D0560987

Destination Wellness

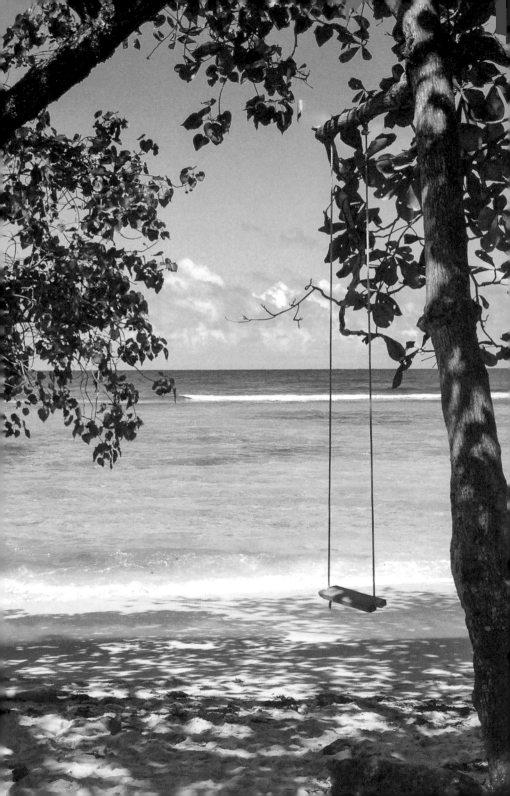

Destination Wellness

GLOBAL SECRETS *for* BETTER LIVING WHEREVER YOU ARE

Annie Daly

CHRONICLE PRISM

Library of Congress Cataloging-in-Publication Data available.
ISBN 978-1-7972-0278-5

Manufactured in China.

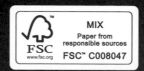

Photographs by Annie Daly. Photograph on page 166
courtesy of Stefanie Kümmerle. Design by Laura Palese.
Typesetting by Happenstance Type-O-Rama. Typeset in Founders
Grotesk, Lulo, Pitch, Sign Painter, and Untitled Serif.

10 9 8 7 6 5 4 3 2 1

Chronicle books and gifts are available at special quantity discounts to
corporations, professional associations, literacy programs, and other
organizations. For details and discount information, please contact our
premiums department at corporatesales@chroniclebooks.com or at
1-800-759-0190.

CHRONICLE PRISM

Chronicle Prism is an imprint of Chronicle Books LLC,
680 Second Street, San Francisco, California 94107

www.chronicleprism.com

FOR RAHUL

YOU ARE THE BEST
LIFE COPILOT
I COULD ASK FOR.

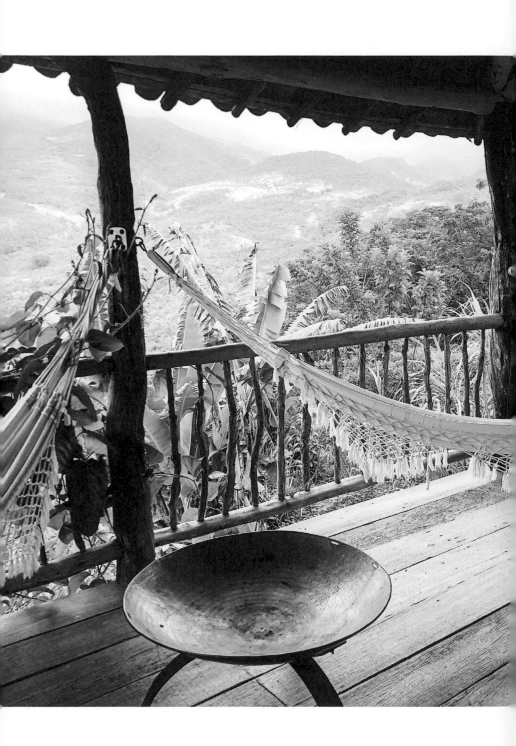

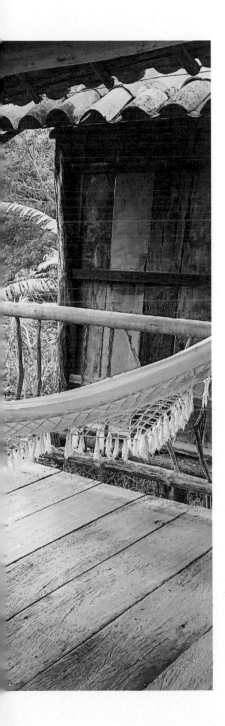

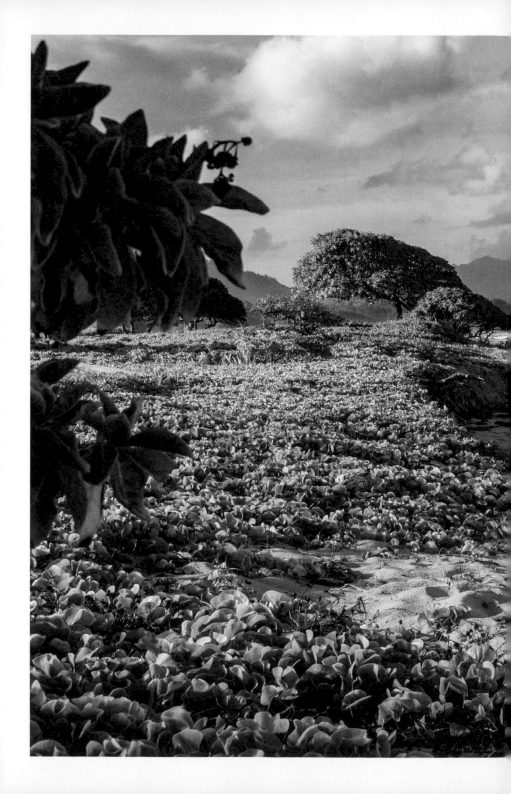

"One's destination is never a place, but a new way of seeing things."

— HENRY MILLER

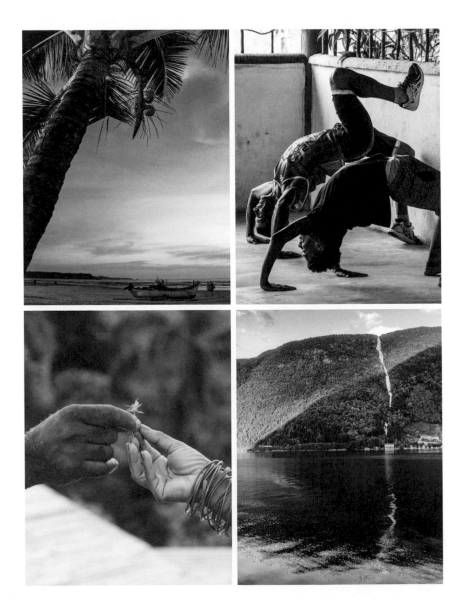

Before
TAKEOFF

*I*T WAS THE "high-vibe" marinara sauce that put me over the edge.

There I was, sitting at my desk at work in downtown Manhattan, sipping my morning coffee, when the email that changed everything arrived in my inbox.

"High-vibe cooking is the new organic," the subject line declared. "It's better for the heart, decreases inflammation, tastes better, and has anti-aging benefits," the email continued, citing no one.

The publicist who wrote the email offered to send me some samples of the sauce, presumably so I could taste some of the "vibes" myself. As an editor at one of the biggest wellness magazines in the country, it was my job to know and report on what's out there, so I accepted the offer. And guess what? When the sauce in question arrived a couple weeks later, I discovered that it was not, as its name may have you believe, packed with vibe-heavy CBD, nor was it blended with some rare strain of mood-enhancing homegrown herbs. Nope, it was just plain old tomato sauce, a big ol' jar of marketing garbage.

Twelve years into my career as a lifestyle journalist, I was used to getting these gimmicky offerings that vowed to lead us all to the wellness promised land. Public relations professionals, eager to get some coverage for the product they're representing, routinely send editors care packages filled with the latest products du jour, "just to get it on our radars." In the months leading up to the high-vibe sauce, I'd also received, in no particular order, "brain dust" delivered in a smooth, pastel-purple sachet bag that promised to "nourish my consciousness from the inside out," a set of chakra-balancing crystals that were guaranteed to help heal my anxiety, and a six-pack of activated charcoal bottled drinks that would allegedly detox me in ways no bottled drink had ever detoxed me before. But even though all of those products were just as bewildering as the sauce, the sauce was my own personal tipping point.

Just days before it had arrived, I'd published an essay about the hypocrisy of the wellness industry, and the essay was still occupying prime real estate on the website and in my head space. In it, I'd written about how my years on staff as a travel journalist had afforded me the privilege of traveling around the world and seeing how other people live, and during that time, I'd noticed that wellness isn't *like* this in many other places around the world.

In New York, I'd gotten into the habit of forking over $36 for a boutique boot camp class, which I could not afford, and buying $12 green smoothies, which at my rate of consumption I *definitely* could not afford. I'd been justifying these purchases by telling myself they were good for my health—and it seemed others were doing the same. I'd watched as people on the Internet had started to purchase $72 healing candles, at first under the vague pretense that they were just "seeing what all of the fuss was about," but eventually without a disclaimer at all.

Meanwhile, on my travels, I'd met Zrinka in Croatia, who takes a dip in the Adriatic Sea every day and swears the daily dose of salt water is her secret to well-being. And I'd met Teddy in Peru, who hikes in the Andes Mountains on the regular and told me that getting in touch with Pachamama—the goddess of nature, or Earth Mother, to the people of the Andes—is what keeps his spirit going. So I asked myself: How were they able to view health in such a non-commercial, more holistic way? Why couldn't I take a cue from them? Why did I think of wellness as such a commodity, when it could be more about my values and the way I live my life?

It was these questions that prompted me to write about the fundamentally backward commodification of wellness in the United States. This was one of those essays that just tumbled out of me one day, where I didn't even have to pause or procrasticlean or refresh Twitter eight million times to get the words out, because it was all so clear: I could not go on like this. I *had* to change. It seemed I had accidentally internalized the idea that self-care was synonymous with self-inflicted debt, but Zrinka and Teddy and countless others were all doing just fine without "purifying" Himalayan salt lamps. Why couldn't I do the same?

My thoughts had resonated with people. Turns out, I wasn't the only one fed up with the state of wellness in America today.

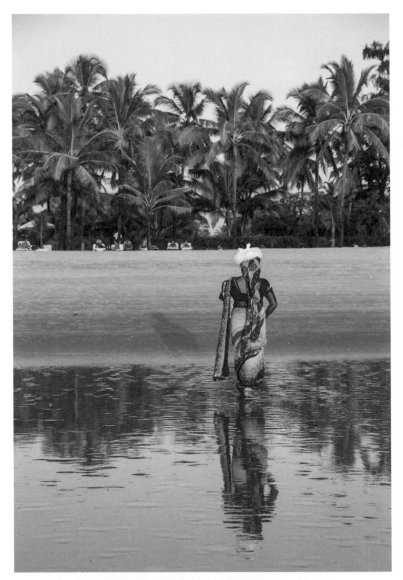

Goa, India: My previous travels around the world had
inspired me to start thinking critically about wellness in America.

People were tired of the industry's expensive products and classes, tired of their message that wellness and being well-off go hand in hand. And I was fed up with the fact that I was professionally entwined with these implications. As the wellness magazine's branded content editor, it was quite literally part of my job to sell those wellness products. (I also wrote non-branded editorial articles, like the one with Zrinka and Teddy.) You know those articles you read that say "sponsored by" or "brought to you by" at the top, and then seem to be regular stories except for a casual mention of a brand in the middle? I wrote those. I'm not throwing any shade at the actual magazine where I worked, because they're definitely out there fighting the good fight, sharing valid and inclusive information. But working there gave me a front-row seat to how the wellness industry's (vegan, gluten-free) sausage is made. And the more I learned, the more frustrated I became.

So when the sauce arrived, I began to hatch a plan. I wanted to show people that it's possible to be well without buying all things wellness—and I had a feeling I could do that by looking further afield for inspiration. After all, if there's one thing my time as a travel writer has taught me, it's that travel truly is the best teacher.

THIS BOOK IS THE RESULT OF MONTHS OF TRAVEL ALL AROUND THE GLOBE. During this time, I interviewed more than one hundred people from various cultures and backgrounds and ethnicities about how they view healthy living.

Now, a few caveats before we go any further: I know that it's impossible to capture the overall scope of a culture in just one trip, or ever, really. My findings are just that: my findings. Also, as a white, upper-middle-class woman, I'd be remiss not to recognize how privileged I am to have been able to travel around the world by myself without being racially profiled or feeling scared or going broke. The majority of the hotels and destinations I visited hosted me because they knew I was writing a book, and for that I am incredibly grateful. Not everyone has the ways and means to travel around the world, and I'm very aware that my profession enabled me to put myself in situations that are not accessible to everyone. I'm also aware of the colonialist undertones that emerge when a white woman brings ideas back from foreign countries. With fourteen years of journalistic experience under my belt, the difference between cultural appreciation and cultural appropriation was top of mind during all of my reporting. Cultural studies professor and scholar Akil Houston, PhD, told me that one of the best ways for journalists to honor the cultures they're covering is to learn about and present the ideas within their proper historical context, and that's what I've done here, to the best of my ability. In that way, I treated my research as one of the greatest responsibilities and gifts of my life.

In what I consider to be the most cosmic of cosmic timing, I traveled to Jamaica, Norway, Hawai'i, Japan, India, and Brazil—quite literally a solo circle around the world—in the months *right before* the COVID-19 pandemic brought travel to a halt. (I know.) The specific reason I chose to travel to each country varies, but my overall "why" was the same: These destinations all seemed to embrace healthy living in a way that differs from the

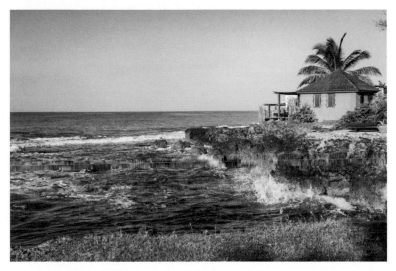

Treasure Beach, Jamaica: Golden light is one of life's best mood boosters.

majority of messages pushed in the wellness industry. Through a combination of reading, talking to friends and family and fellow travel writers, and my own past adventures, I landed on these locations because they were all home to a lifestyle philosophy that piqued my curiosity, one that I hoped could teach me how to think in a different way. I still can't get over the timely fate of it all—especially because the lessons I gathered in those places have taken on even more meaning in the aftermath of "The Great Pause."

THROUGH MY TRAVELS, I LEARNED THAT, GENER-ALLY SPEAKING, WELLNESS IS NOT ABOUT ADDING — IT'S ABOUT SUBTRACTING. It's about stripping yourself down to your core. In the early days of COVID-19, there were all sorts of think pieces floating around about how humanity *needed* this stillness, how it was the universe's way of telling us to slow down. Unfortunately, it took tremendous loss and trauma as a global community to make that happen—to force us to pause and reevaluate our lives—and I can only hope that some of that reflection sticks around in the coming years. But we've needed to slow down and reflect for a good long while now, to stop filling our voids with material possessions and running around in a frenzy. It's just that now this message is even more urgent.

MY TRAVELS TOOK ME THROUGH SOME OF THE LARGEST CITIES AND THE SMALLEST COUNTRYSIDE VILLAGES IN THE WORLD. One of the biggest lessons I learned on the road, a lesson that was prevalent across nearly all cultures and backgrounds and is more timely now than ever before, is that most of us have the things we need already—and we've had them all along. This is especially true for indigenous cultures around the globe, whose ancestors were able to survive on the land for thousands upon thousands of years using only their own wisdom.

Our modern-day problem, of course, is that we've become so far removed from those ancient lessons that we're spinning ourselves in circles, frazzled and confused. Thanks to our phones and our laptops and our pills and our Netflix-and-chills, everything is always buzzing, including our brains. We've created a giant hole between the way it was and the way it is now. And guess what? We're filling that hole with products. The wellness industrial complex is "rescuing" us from our self-induced modern buzz with all sorts of lotions and potions and Lulus and woo-woos that promise to help us feel more grounded and whole. According to the Global Wellness Institute, a nonprofit research and educational resource for the wellness industry, America is the number one "wellness nation" in the entire world, meaning

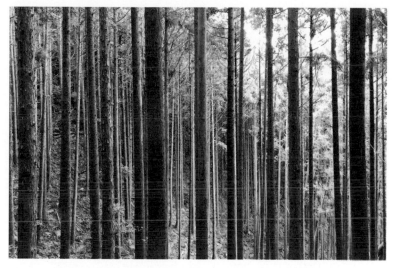

Kumano Kodo, Japan: The stillness of the Japanese forests
helped soothe my buzzing brain.

we're the top spender on wellness. We quite literally buy into the hype the most.

But the products we're buying are coming up empty—and *we're* coming up empty, too. The 2019 annual *World Happiness Report,* published by the United Nations, found that "the years since 2010 have not been good ones for happiness and well-being among Americans." Despite shelling out more and more cash on all things wellness, and despite a general uptick in our standard of living, we're not actually any healthier today than we were in the past. In fact, in many ways, we're less healthy. "This is the Easterlin paradox," the UN report continues. "As the standard of living improves, so should happiness—but it has not." A new report from well-being expert Meik Wiking's Happiness Research Institute aptly refers to this paradox as the "decoupling of wealth and well-being."

I am in no way proposing that this book is going to be our societal quick fix, the magical thing that is going to solve the complicated, twisted wellness paradox in this country. For starters, there *is* no societal quick fix (and I'd argue that our cultural obsession with seeking them out helped get us here in the first place). A person's well-being is only in part a result of their choices, and those choices are inscribed by societal circumstances they often can't control. We have a long way to go to solve the problematic social policies and systemic injustices that are causing much of our stress in the first place. But to the extent that we can effect change in our lives by changing our behaviors, the message I heard on my travels was loud and clear: True well-being is about ditching all of the extras, and looking back to move forward. It's about coming back to our essence. Back to the basics.

It took an around-the-world trip to help me realize that the wellness philosophies that work best are most often the simple ones, the timeless ones that have been around for ages, the ones that are so ingrained in global history, humans around the world have been doing them all along. In fact, much of the health and wellness wisdom in these pages was passed down through oral storytelling, documented not in a scientific, peer-reviewed journal but in the hearts and souls of its messengers. And I'll be honest: I struggled with this idea at first. Absorbing these philosophical, sometimes-amorphous concepts requires a particular type of loose, open-minded thinking that may not come 100 percent naturally to all Westerners—it certainly didn't come naturally to me. I started out my career as a health reporter for national magazines, so I've been trained from the get-go to find proof in the form of evidence-based, complete, randomized scientific studies published in peer-reviewed journals. This is how we do health in the West, and this is especially how I was taught to cover it as a reporter. I will never not hear my first fact-checker's voice in my head: *Where's the proof?*

But the more I chatted with people all over the world who follow the ancient wisdom of their ancestors, the more I realized that there are other ways to interpret and understand well-being. The proof is in the history. Many of the lessons in this book have helped people live well for thousands of years, and now it's on us to get back to those fundamentals, to set up our lives with the things that have always made existence healthy and enjoyable, but somehow managed to slip away when the modern world took over: Human connection. Mother Earth. Whole foods. Soul.

LISTEN: THERE'S A LOT TO BE ANGRY ABOUT IN THE WORLD TODAY. That's partly why the wellness industry is thriving. Products like essential-oil diffusers and pricey bath bombs offer a temporary and soothing solution to frustrating issues that are so far out of our control. But there is a difference between "self-soothing" and "self-care." While products that may calm us in the moment are often labeled as *self-care*, they are merely an emotional Band-Aid. True self-care lies in the deep work. The soul work.

I will be the first to admit that I am not going to abandon all boutique fitness classes for the rest of time, and that I will continue to buy too-expensive smoothies and serums here and there

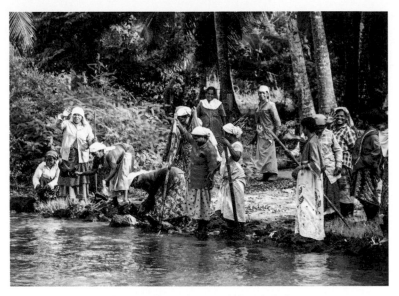

Kerala, India: Watching other people live their lives opens the door to examining your own.

during treat-yourself moments. After all, when you take those things for exactly what they are—a fun way to get moving and motivated; an afternoon boost when you're feeling sluggish— they can work just fine. But the problem comes when we expect those fancy classes and products to be *more* than what they are. The problem comes when we expect them to *solve* us, to *heal* us, to help us achieve a deep sense of well-being, when that's not what they're for. Self-care as we know it today was never supposed to be about the $100 candles. Originally created by and for Black people during the civil rights movement in the 1960s, self-care was always bigger than that. It was a political act, a way for marginalized groups to make it through in a world that's working against them. Thanks to capitalism, it has morphed into a commercial enterprise, but let's be clear: True well-being is not something you can buy. It's about tapping into what's inside of you already. An amethyst crystal–infused water bottle will not help you do that. But I'm hopeful that these healthy-living philosophies will.

We travel to witness and to learn about other ways of doing things, other ways of living. Seeing how different people go about their days makes it easier to reflect on our own. When I'm home in New York, I often get stuck in my own thought patterns, wondering what I'll eat for breakfast and when I will do my laundry and if that thing I wrote was actually good and which route I will take to the dinner I'm going to that night. But travel forces me to get outside of my own head. If nothing else, it's an epic reminder to think bigger, to remember that my way is not the only way.

Of course, I'm aware that it's not possible to apply all of the lessons in this book to your own life. The people I interviewed live *there* and you live *here*, and with that comes a whole host of logistical complications. It's hard to soothe yourself with a swim in the ocean every day like many Hawaiians do, for example, if you don't live near a body of water. But if there's one lesson I want you to take away from this journey, it's that weaving these ideas into your life is a revolution of the mind, more than anything else. And as it happens, your mind can live anywhere you want.

xx Annie

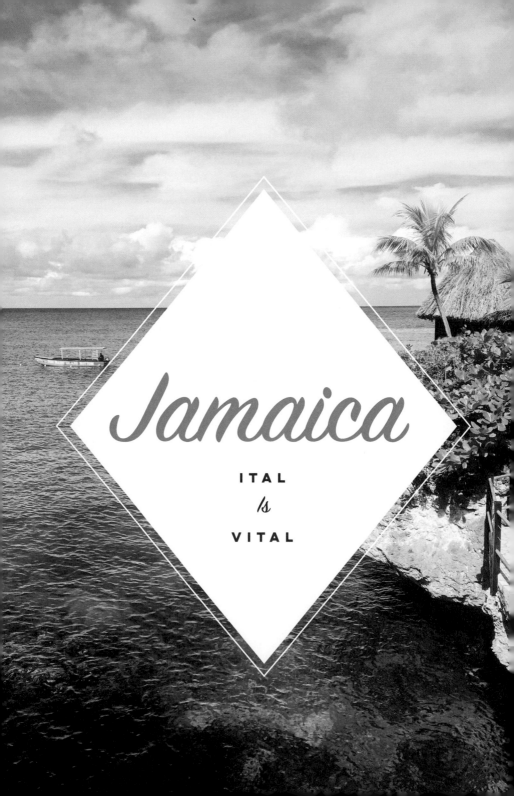

Jamaica

ITAL
Is
VITAL

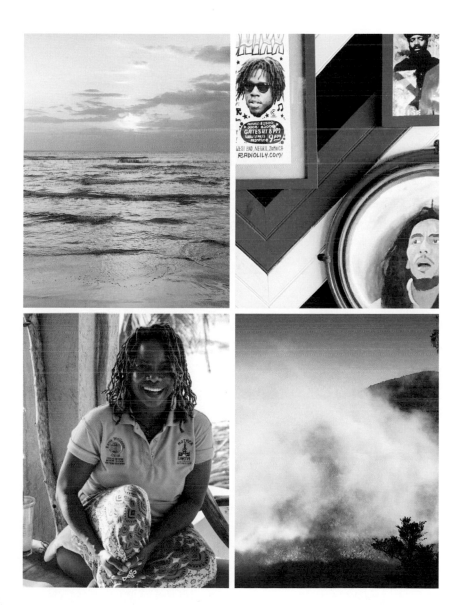

*H*AVE YOU EVER noticed how in magazine profiles, the celebrities always seem to have just "stepped out" from someplace cool, or seem to "waltz in" looking effortlessly chic, wearing "down-to-earth" clothes like fresh-pressed jeans and a breezy white T-shirt? I always thought those phrases were a cop-out, something lazy writers say when they don't know what else to say, but I am here to tell you that they are not. On the day I interviewed Chronixx, a popular Rastafari reggae star from Jamaica, for the wellness magazine, he really *did* waltz into the Jamaican restaurant in Manhattan where I was meeting him for the first time. At home in New York, most people I know are more likely to hurl themselves into a place full throttle, a bundle of energy and nerves, but Chronixx had a nice little spring in his step. He looked genuinely happy to be alive in that moment, a refreshing change of pace from the usual New York frenzy.

"So, have you checked out any yoga classes while you've been here in New York?" I asked him once we'd settled into a quiet vinyl booth tucked into the back of the restaurant. As a longtime fan, I was pumped and a little bit nervous to get the opportunity to chat with him about his take on wellness. I knew that most Rastafari—which is both the social and political movement that originated in Jamaica, and the name for the people who follow it—have a generally healthy outlook on the world, and I thought my admittedly light question may help us ease into a conversation about his. But Chronixx did not need to dip his toe in first. "Nah, yoga is not an event," he replied. "It's not something that you have to *go* to."

I looked at him, a bit confused. His music rep had emailed me a few weeks earlier, after she saw that I retweet Chronixx on Twitter all the time. "You're one of the only mainstream wellness journalists who's also a Chronixx fan, and he's super into health and well-being, so I thought his views could be a unique angle for you," she'd written. I could've sworn she said he was a yogi, too.

"Oh, so you're not into yoga?" I asked. "I definitely thought you were."

"No, no, I do yoga every day, just a pose or two, mostly just stretches as soon as I wake up," Chronixx clarified. "But I don't do a thirty- or sixty-minute routine or anything like that. For me, yoga isn't about the physical poses. It's about the spiritual practice. The mental yoga."

He had a point. Yoga isn't something you have to *go* to—it can live in all of us, all of the time, if we think of it that way. Why hadn't I ever heard anyone put it like that before? I was so used to my fellow New Yorkers scurrying around, yoga mats in tow, stressing out about being late to relax. I thought of all the trendy classes I got invitations to attend as part of my job—dog yoga, namaste rosé yoga, hip-hop yoga—and they suddenly seemed so over the top, not to mention a far cry from yoga's cultural roots in India. I told Chronixx he had inspired me to look at well-being through a wider lens already.

"To be healthy is to create a better Earth," he nodded, carrying on with his trademark philosophical spirit. "And that's why I eat an Ital diet, too."

At that point, I had a basic understanding that Ital, derived from the word *vital*, is the plant-based lifestyle that most Rastas embrace. (Followers of the Rastafari movement are also referred to as Rastas or Rastafarians.) As a devoted lifelong fan of reggae—the music deeply associated with Rastafari—I'd heard the word in countless songs over the years, from Damian Marley's "Born to Be Wild," in which he sings about having an "Ital vision," to Bunny Wailer's "Cool Runnings," where he repeats that his "riddim is Ital" over and over again. But perhaps more important, I'd also learned about Ital firsthand on my first trip to Jamaica a couple years back. My now-husband Rahul and I had booked a room at a Rastafari guesthouse called Jah B's after we discovered that we'd both grown up listening to reggae and were increasingly curious about the culture that had shaped the music that defined our youth. Located high up in the Blue Mountains, about a two-hour drive from Kingston, the guesthouse was an incredible window into Rastafari culture. On our first morning there, Jah B himself—a Rasta farmer and business owner who grows all of his own food—had cooked us a homemade Ital breakfast, with scrambled ackee (a tropical fruit that sort of looks like egg when cooked), homegrown tomatoes, Scotch bonnet peppers, a local leafy green called *callaloo*, and fresh Blue Mountain coffee straight from the source.

"Our bodies are all we have, so we have to nourish them wisely," he'd told us as he set down our plates and pointed to his huge compost bin piled high with plantain peels and mango skins. It was still early, around 9 a.m. or so, and the Blue Mountains were bathed in buttery morning light so golden, even the compost pile looked beautiful. Jah B had continued to tell us about his homegrown lifestyle, about how it's our duty as humans to protect our bodies, and how he's dedicated his life to living naturally in the hills because, to him, it's the only way to live.

When you mention Rastafari in casual conversation, many people immediately picture those red, yellow, and green crocheted caps with long dreads, or a bag of fresh ganja. But the truth is that Rastafari has gotten appropriated around the world. Sadly, people often think of Rastafarians as lazy stoners who sit around blazing weed on the beach all day, but there was Jah B, a captivating, health-minded business owner, telling us about how he's out there on his farm day in and day out, growing his own food to nourish his body and spirit. I wanted to shout his wisdom from the rooftops. Jah B had even taught us a bit about the loose meaning of Ital itself: Though there isn't a universally agreed-upon definition of the philosophy, and all Rastas interpret it slightly differently, the majority believe that its main goal is to enhance your vitality through the food you eat. That often includes avoiding animal products, processed foods, and additives, and growing your own food as much as possible—all core tenets of Jah B's day-to-day lifestyle.

Back on that trip, Rahul and I had gone hiking in the Blue Mountains after breakfast, and we'd packed up the next day to

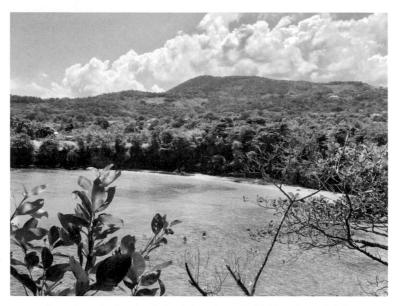

Port Antonio: On cloud nine in Portie, still thinking about Jah B.

head to Port Antonio, a lush, laid-back beach town on the north-east coast of the island. In "Portie," as the locals call it, we'd had a grand old Jamaican time, drinking loads of white rum and Red Stripe, eating the juiciest jerk chicken, and playing around in the turquoise waters of the Blue Lagoon, a deep, spring-fed natural pool surrounded by mangroves and massive banyan trees. But even though we'd spent our next days soaking up lots of sun and lots of rum—not exactly an Ital move—we hadn't stopped think-ing about Jah B. I kept imagining what his place might look like if it were in America: a boutique hotel marketed loudly as "healthy" and "vegan," heralding its "locally sourced" food and surely charging premium prices. The real Jah B's was a glimpse into what genuine well-being could look like without commodifying its essence. And sitting there years later chatting with Chronixx, who had just shared similar anti-commercialism sentiments with me, my initial time at Jah B's came flooding back into focus.

That's why, when the time came to pick where to go for this book, I chose to head back to Jamaica—this time to the other side of the island to check out some other Rastafari farms I'd been hearing about. Ital seemed to hold the true key to eating and living well, and I wanted to know more.

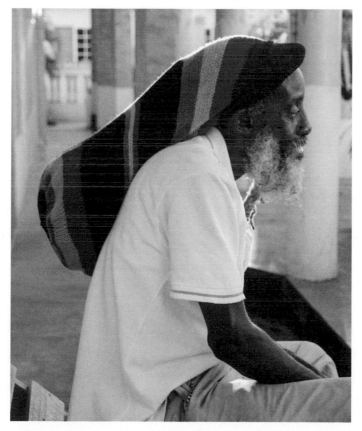

Treasure Beach: Don't you want to know what he's thinking about?

The History of Rastafari

It's impossible to talk about Ital without first placing it in the full context of Rastafari, as it's a big part of the larger movement. While Rastafari began in Jamaica's most impoverished communities in the 1930s, its roots can be traced back to the beginning of the trans-Atlantic slave trade. Here's a brief—but by no means conclusive—overview:

1600 TO 1900: Between ten and twelve million Africans were captured in dehumanizing slave raids and transported across the Atlantic Ocean. The British (who ruled Jamaica until 1962) transported over one million Africans to the island to work on sugar plantations as enslaved people.

LATE 1800s: Displaced Africans discovered multiple references to Ethiopia in the Holy Bible. This gave rise to the redemptive tradition known as *Ethiopianism*, in which some people of the African diaspora identified with Ethiopia-Africa as their homeland.

1914: Jamaican political leader Marcus Garvey started the Universal Negro Improvement Association, whose mission was to end European colonization and reunite the diaspora with their original homeland, and, thus, their physical, cultural, and spiritual freedom. In the late 1920s, Garvey encouraged his followers to "Look to Africa, for the day of deliverance is near."

1930: A young Ethiopian prince, Ras Tafari Makonnen, was crowned His Imperial Majesty, Emperor Haile Selassie I, Emperor of Ethiopia. He took the title King of Kings, Lord of Lords, Conquering Lion of the Tribe of Judah, and, interpreting these as the titles reserved for the Second Coming of Christ, a number of preachers in Jamaica began to preach the divinity of Ras Tafari. The goal of all Rastafari from that day forward was to align themselves culturally, spiritually, and physically with the Emperor and his kingdom. This thinking went against that of mainstream Jamaican society, which was still ruled by the British colonialists.

1934: Leonard Howell, the first person in Jamaica to preach Rastafari, was arrested, tried, and convicted for sedition. This was the first of many examples of Rastas being shunned by Jamaican society.

1935: Italy invaded Ethiopia on October 3. The Second Italo-Ethiopian War lasted until May 1936, when Italy occupied Ethiopia. The war became a rallying cry and led to a worldwide mobilization in support of the Ethiopian cause, which was central to the emergence of the Rastafari movement.

1940: Leonard Howell established Pinnacle, the first Rastafari commune in Jamaica. The commune attracted more than one thousand followers who engaged in farming and ganja cultivation. It was raided by the government several times in the early 1940s, and again in 1954, which dispersed the majority of Howell's followers to the slums of Kingston.

EARLY 1950s: Rastafari in the ghettos and shanty towns of Kingston began to create a distinctive culture through which they identified as Ethiopians and spiritually aligned with Jah Rastafari (a term for Emperor Haile Selassie I). These cultural practices, referred to as *livity* (life force), were used to separate them from the oppressive society they called Babylon. In the mid-to-late 1950s, they developed Ital as one such practice, meant to sanctify the body as the Temple of Jah.

1963: Just one year after Jamaican independence, the government rounded up and tortured hundreds of Rastas and killed an unknown number in what's known as the Coral Gardens Incident. Rastas then fled to the hills of Jamaica, where many—but not all—live today.

1966: Emperor Haile Selassie I visited Jamaica, a true watershed moment in the history of the Rasta movement and Jamaican society. The government underestimated Rastafari's influence, and its leaders were surprised when an estimated one hundred thousand Rastafari showed up to welcome the Emperor at the airport. At a formal state ceremony, the Emperor awarded gold medals to thirteen Rasta leaders, thus elevating Rastafari to Jamaica's national stage for the first time.

1970s: Reggae music emerged due in large part to the global popularity of Bob Marley and the Wailers. Reggae and its powerful messages of past oppression, peaceful resistance, and future unity began to spread around the world—and it's one of the most well-known musical genres today.

I'd heard about the farm through the grapevine, how the owners were doing cool things up there in the hills, and the moment my taxi driver dropped me off at their homestead, I could tell the whispers were true. Run by plant-loving couple Chris Binns (a Rasta farmer) and Lisa Binns (a gourmet chef), Stush in the Bush is the type of place you dream of moving to when you dream of moving off grid. Their cozy homestead, built with all-local wood, is perched on the top of a hillside overlooking groves of coconut trees. It made me feel more eco-conscious just by looking at it, with a big open-air deck and giant windows that let in the light. (*Stush*, of Stush in the Bush, means "stylish" in the local patois.) Although they're only 40 miles from touristy Montego Bay, the farm feels far away from the modern world in both distance and years, a place where time stands still and the only noise is the sound of the birds and the breeze rustling through the trees.

Lisa brought out fresh coconut waters when I arrived, and we all sat out on the deck to chat. "I'm excited to discuss Ital with you," Chris began, "especially because Ital was [one of] the original vegan [diets]. It's great that the rest of the world seems to be finally catching up." He was barefoot, wearing jeans and a white shirt, and had his long dreadlocks—often referred to as just locs—wrapped up in a bun. (Rastafari grow dreadlocks as a representation of their natural selves, far from Babylonian influence.) "I think we are all rediscovering what it means to be a part of nature as a whole," he reflected. "This generation now is recognizing that our way of living, especially in our relationship to nature, is not sustainable."

After a little more back and forth on global warming and the scary future of our planet—standard topics when you are interviewing farmers, I've learned—we got to the point. "Ital is rooted in this basis of removing yourself from all things artificial and immersing yourself in nature as the foundation for absolutely everything," Chris explained. "And a big reason for that is that Rastas were shunned. Oppressed. They were in the hills, or in the gulleys, or in the ghettos, having been chased from the cities for their beliefs. And when they were separated, they had to actually produce their own food, so most Rastas planted something. Once they did that, they developed a connection to where their food was coming from. I would say that to this day, most Rastas still plant something or know someone who does plant."

Chris and Lisa are definitely planters themselves. Back in 2009, Lisa—who was born in Barbados but raised in Brooklyn—came to Jamaica on vacation and met Chris at a friend's gathering in Portland, a parish on the island's northeast coast. In a movie-meets-real-life moment, they locked eyes from across the room and were married two months later. According to Chris, Lisa brought the stush to the bush when she moved in, and now they practice regenerative agriculture to grow an abundance of crops on their farm, from breadfruit trees to sweet potatoes to herbs like oregano and cilantro. They also hold events for travelers and locals alike, like twinkly-light outdoor dinners that begin with a tour of the farm. When we had lunch outside later on, they served up a truly farm-to-table spread of crispy fried green plantains dipped in homemade chimichurri sauce, followed by wood-fired basil pesto pizzas prepared in their stone-cut open-air grill. We toasted with glasses of a fresh batch of passion fruit livity juice.

Toward the end of our lunch, I began to think about my own (poor) connection to food and to the land. I'd just eaten one of the tastiest meals of my life, made tastier by the knowledge that I was sitting on the land it came from. But let's be real: In my life in NYC, I was all too quick to open up a bag of the latest organic, plant-based paleo puffs and call it dinner. Back at the wellness magazine, I was constantly trying out trendy new "wellness" snacks from the "free table" in our office, and as a freelancer, publicists simply sent the snacks straight to my apartment door. I knew, deep down, that they weren't exactly healthy, but they were so easy, so available, and I didn't really think of them as unhealthy, either. I tended to just eat what was around, whatever I could get my hands on that seemed healthy enough at the time. But chatting with Lisa and Chris and then enjoying their delicious food helped me realize that my reliance on commercialized wellness wasn't going to lead me to a place of true well-being.

"We Rastas like to say that 'Ital is vital,' but we're not just talking about the food—Ital is more about the lifestyle," Chris continued. "It's about choosing to unplug from some of the trappings of modern society. Ital is ultimately a way to break free of Babylon by living on your own terms like Rastas originally did in the hills. And a big part of that is a respect for the environment and for what Mother Nature brings to you."

How Rastafari Arrived at Ital from Vital (and How You Can Elevate Your Speech)

These days, the phrase "set your intention" is a wellness buzzword. Yet its message has always been a core part of how Rastafarians speak. They created their own language with the intention to take back the power from their oppressors in daily life. This language, sometimes referred to as *Ivar, Iyaric,* or *I-talk,* is based around the concept of *wordsound,* which is defined by a conscious use of sound.

Rastafari language emphasizes equality through the concept of "I," Jah Rastafari (God). Rastas believe that everyone exists as one person unified by Jah. They reject any separation between "you and me." For this reason, Rastas choose to begin many words with "I." In addition to changing "vital" to "Ital," they also say "I-nity" instead of "unity." Rastas also say "I and I" in place of "we," to reflect the idea that we (I and I) all embody the Divine—and we should all love each other like we love ourselves.

Rastas also observe a deep African tradition in which words are understood to carry positive and negative vibrations. The belief is that negative sounds reflect their oppression, whereas positive sounds spread their values of peace and love—so they carefully scrutinize words to eliminate and/or replace negative sounds. Check out these examples, and consider your own word choices. Are there any you could swap for something more positive?

enjoy > fulljoy
(they do not want the joy to end)

appreciate > apprecilove
(they do not feel the vibration of hate)

understand > overstand
(one should not stand under an idea)

conversation > reasoning
(they do not sit down to chat with the intention to con anyone)

hello > yes I ("hell" and "low" both sound negative, whereas "yes I" is uplifting)

birthday > Earthstrong
(to keep the connection with Mother Earth)

Veganism often elicits a strong reaction in people, especially those who don't see a problem with eating meat. "Oh, those vegans," the naysayers sigh, "up on their high horse about not eating animal products." Research has shown that there are benefits to following a well-planned vegan diet, but the longer I hung out with Chris and Lisa, the more I realized that that wasn't even the entire point. The point is that Rastafari who interpret the Ital diet strictly do it out of a pure, genuine love for Mother Nature and a desire to live on their own terms, not just for health reasons and not to spite those who don't follow suit. It's as much a matter of cultural principles as it is a matter of health.

While I tend to forget that Mother Nature did not *bring me* the activated superfood popcorn on the free table at work, Rastafari are very clear about the idea that she's the one in charge. Not us, not the delivery guy, and certainly not the free table. Everything we ate, minus the pizza dough, had come from their farm, because Mother Nature is the one who does the bringing. She comes first, and we are secondary. It's a beautiful sentiment, this idea that Mother Nature's the one in charge. And that's what Chris and Lisa were ultimately getting at:

THE STORY OF ITAL IS THE STORY OF HOW AN ENTIRE WELLNESS MOVEMENT ROSE FROM OPPRESSION.

After my trip, I called up Jahlani Niaah, PhD, one of the foremost Rastafari scholars in the world, to chat about what I'd learned on my travels. As a cultural and Rastafari studies professor at the University of the West Indies in Jamaica, Dr. Niaah— who goes by Jahlani in conversations with journalists—is also

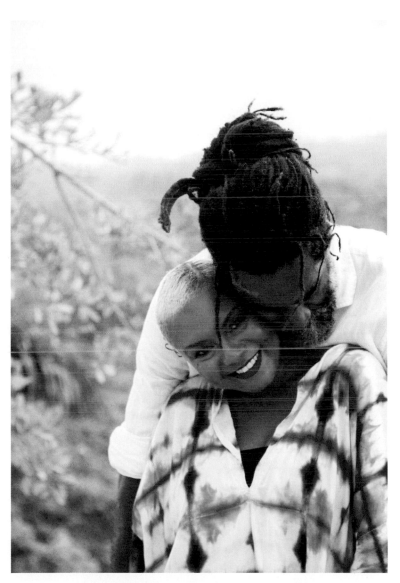

Free Hill: Stush in the Bush's Chris and Lisa Binns
share a hug at home on the farm.

the author of many Rastafari books, including *Let Us Start with Africa: Foundations of Rastafari Scholarship*. Like Chris, he pointed out that Ital was initially a reaction to Babylon—the Rastafari term for anything related to colonialism—but then emerged into its own plant-focused lifestyle as a result.

"At first, Ital was the resistance ethos undertaken by enslaved people in Jamaica, a political critique that anchored its wellness on a rejection of certain kinds of unsustainable imports—like salt and cured meats—that Rastafari linked to the lifestyle diseases coming out of colonialism," he told me. "But this conversation eventually strengthened into the philosophy of a plant-based diet. And this plant-based diet became increasingly understood as a way of liberating oneself by engaging in a pragmatic self-reliance that included responsibility over your own wellness," he continued.

Spend enough time with Rastafari, and this idea of viewing your diet as a political act, as a way to maintain self-reliance in the face of historical oppression, will continue to come up again and again. After Stush in the Bush, I visited a farm east of Negril called Zimbali Retreats, where the owners, Alecia and Mark Swainbank, who are both Rastafari, even told me that they have a self-reliance life motto on their farm: Carry your own water. "What that means is, go to the stream to get the water if you can, so you know where your food and drink come from," Mark explained one afternoon during my visit.

Mark and Alecia created Zimbali as a symbol of their mutual dedication to Mother Earth. I arrived at the 7.5-acre farm early one morning after a bumpy ride through jungly, rocky, vine-tangled hills, but despite my lingering post-ride nausea, I felt a sense of calm wash over me as I got out of the car and looked around. There were a few bright red hibiscus plants by the wooden gate, but otherwise, it was just . . . green. I'm talking jungle green, luscious green, the kind of green that smells like it's just rained even when it hasn't. Mark and Alecia came to the door offering up a plate of freshly cut cucumbers drizzled in homemade coconut oil and sprinkled with sea salt, plus a cup of magenta sorrel (Jamaican hibiscus) juice.

The snack, sourced entirely from their farm out back, *tasted* like Jamaica. And that was their whole thing: Everything tasted like Jamaica because everything was *from* Jamaica. Alecia, a Rastafari from birth, grew up in the hills directly around Zimbali. It was all right there. One afternoon during my stay, I went for a hike deep into the mountains to visit Fiyah, a Rasta farmer who works on their farm, at his two-floor treehouse with sweeping views of the mountains below. Over an open-air fire pit, he prepared an Ital stew straight from his personal farm, with potatoes, cassava, plantains, and more. "Nothing is artificial in this meal, and that's how it goes with the Rastaman and Rastawoman," he told me as he placed a pile of local goodness on my plate.

Touring the rest of the Zimbali land during my stay, I spotted all sorts of tropical fruits and vegetables and healing plants. I saw *Cymbopogon* (lemongrass), which is used to help muscle pain. One of the farmers told me that the bright red and orange flowers from their *Spathodea* (African tulip tree) make the best natural eye drops ever. I saw *Morinda citrifolia* (noni plant), which can help with inflammation, infections, and high blood pressure, and is also a great addition to smoothies for an antioxidant boost. Most of all, I saw a backyard grocery store and hospital all in one. "When you get your own water from the stream, or your own food from your farm, you see your connection to Mother Nature," Alecia emphasized. "And we believe that actually seeing where your food comes from inspires you to keep living as naturally as you can. My health is my wealth, and if you really see your health as your wealth, too, then you're going to try to protect your health in every way you can."

OF COURSE, AS A THIRTY-SOMETHING WOMAN WHO LIVES IN BROOKLYN, NEW YORK, I DON'T EXACTLY LIVE FROM THE LAND MYSELF.

I admire all of the Rastafari I chatted with in Jamaica for creating their own self-reliant world, and I often fantasize about making a similar move myself. Who hasn't watched *Planet Earth* or *Tiny House Nation* and dreamed of packing it all in to live in harmony with nature? For years I've daydreamed of starting a new life with kale beds and a babbling brook in my backyard, and it doesn't help that Rahul likes to entertain these daydreams as well. We've spent too many Saturdays scrolling through StreetEasy, scoping out farms in upstate New York and wondering *what if?* But in the end, we both ultimately come back to the fact that we are too invested in our home in New York City to uproot ourselves in such an epic way right now. Our friends are here, our careers are here, and despite our wandering minds, we actually really *like* it here. And so, for better or for worse, we are part of the very commercialism that Rastas are up against— which is why I decided to seek out some Rastafari when I was back home in NYC. I wanted to see how they make it work in the urban jungle despite the clear lack of banana trees and fresh sorrel.

New York has a large Caribbean community, so it didn't take me long to find a good source: an Ital restaurant in Brooklyn called Ital Kitchen. When I arrived for lunch with the

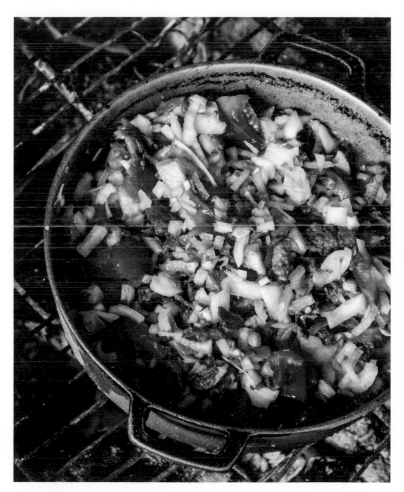

Negril: Fiyah's nourishing Ital stew, heating up high in the mountains.

restaurant's owner, Michael Gordon, a couple days after I'd gotten home, it was a cold day in Brooklyn, and I was excited to get a taste and feel of the tropics again. Although I hadn't even been home for a week, I'd already hopped right back into my urban grind, with the wine nights and the workout classes and the subway grime and the waiting time, and I was even more curious than ever about how to maintain an Ital ethos in the big city.

Michael met me at the door and told me that I was just in time: He was in the middle of cooking up a "nice little Ital stew" back in the kitchen. I'd arrived an hour before his restaurant opened, so we had the place to ourselves, and the cold melted away as soon as I entered the room. The walls were painted in warm tones, mostly oranges, magentas, and greens, and there were houseplants everywhere. Michael had Peter Tosh playing softly in the background, and I could smell the stew, with notes of ginger and fresh thyme, simmering on the stove. Even though the traffic and the horns and the buzz were all just outside the door, they felt very far away.

"How do you follow Ital principles when you're here in Brooklyn, away from fresh farmland?" I asked him once we'd sat down at the table and started to dig into our stews. They were piping hot, made with potatoes, spinach, onions, vegetable broth, and fresh herbs. Simple yet delicious.

Michael, who grew up in Jamaica before moving to New York, took a deep breath before he began. "Ital isn't just about food, and it's not just about the farming, either," he said, echoing the various sentiments I'd heard in Jamaica. "So much of Ital farming, in its earliest stages, was as much about the *idea* that you could plant your own food as it was about the planting itself.

The *idea* that you could separate yourself from society came first, and the planting was almost secondary," he explained. And it's that idea, more than anything else, that Michael carries into his life as a Brooklyn-based Rastafari, though he does have more tangible tips, too.

Planting something is a good place to start, even if it's just a small seedling that you take care of on your window. "Americans tend to get plants that don't grow things, but what's the point?" he laughed. "Watching something go through an amazing period of growth in such a short period of time is really powerful, especially when you can see and eat the fruits of your labor. It'll help you feel more connected to nature, and remember that we are all one with this Earth." Surrounding yourself with plants at home also helps create what Michael refers to as a "bubble of vibes," aka your own little urban oasis sanctuary. "City life is hard, with everyone rushing around doing things, so you have to just build your own little world with your plants and your music and your cooking," he said as I nodded my head *yes yes yes*. I am a firm believer in the magic of house vibes. For me, that means filling my apartment with green plants and cozy twinkly lights, lighting incense and crisp white candles, and turning on uplifting music—usually reggae, let's be honest—as soon as I walk in the door.

Cooking your own non-processed meals is another way to break free of commercialism and maintain self-reliance. "Everyone always asks me if my restaurant is on Seamless, and I say to them, 'Of course not!'" Michael laughed. "Americans always want everything so quick, but I want everyone to take the time to cook for themselves if they are going to eat at home," he said. "Sometimes Americans try to complicate things with all of the processed foods and the delivery meals and eating on the go. But your health is the one thing you have control over, so why not take advantage of that and make sure you are eating the most natural foods you can?"

Of course, not all people *do* have control over their health. Those with chronic illnesses struggle to control their own bodies, for example. And access to fresh food is a huge problem in America, as is the luxury of time and money to seek it out and prepare it. That said, if you do have access to fresh foods, it may be easier than you think to incorporate them into your daily life. If you can, Michael suggests joining a co-op to cut costs. He grows lots of fresh herbs and vegetables in his backyard herb garden during the warmer months, but during the rest of the year, he gets all of his food at the Park Slope Food Coop. "Organic food is so expensive, so you've gotta belong to something, be a part of something, to be able to afford it," he said as I was slurping up the last of my stew. While membership to most co-ops depends on putting in work hours every few weeks, doing so gives you access to the best produce from local farmers—and a discount on your food. To Michael, joining one is a no-brainer, an ideal way to ensure that he's choosing non-processed, whole, plant-based foods.

What he's ultimately getting at, though—what all of the Rastafarian men and women in Jamaica I spoke with were getting at—is that Ital is ultimately about self-reliance. And self-reliance takes effort. Self-reliance is about showing up for your co-op shift, even when it's inconvenient, and making the time to cook for yourself as much as you can, even when you feel lazy. Perhaps most importantly, it's about trusting nature to give you what you need, not multinational corporations or even smaller businesses that use overly processed ingredients. And isn't that the whole thing? The original Rastafari believed that treating their bodies well would bring them closer to Jah Rastafari, so they did everything in their power to make that happen—and they still do today. I hung out with a Rastafari woman named Empress Thandi in Treasure Beach, a laid-back town all the way in the south of Jamaica, who runs a healing center called the Rasta Wellness Centre with its own take-out food shop, Ital Mama Cafe. Empress Thandi—known simply as "Empress" around Treasure Beach—reminded me that "honoring her body temple" does take effort, but in the end, it's always worth it.

"Fresh food has a different kind of vibration, a different kind of frequency," she explained one afternoon as we were looking out over the ocean. "See that coconut tree right there? It's pulling up water from the ocean and still able to give you alkaline water. So, to me, wellness is about honoring that," she told me. "It's about making sure that everything we're doing, we're honoring that which is in a natural state." You're not going to find wellness in that bottle of $8 processed juice with added adaptogens. You're going to find it by honoring the natural world and by putting in the effort to connect to your food in a deeper way.

When I first came to Jamaica with Rahul, I was mostly in it for the music. We had decided to start our trip in the Blue Mountains not just because of the nature or the hiking but also

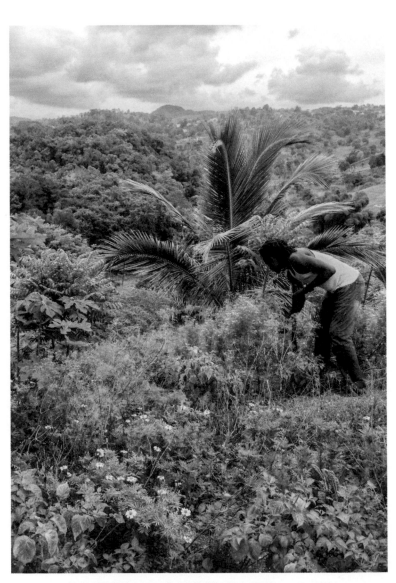

**Free Hill: Raise your hand if this photo makes you want
to live a more natural lifestyle.**

because both of us had a reggae song we wanted to sing while we were there. (I know: I found my do-it-for-the-song soulmate.)

Rahul grew up loving the folk song "Jamaica Farewell," which instilled in him a deep desire to explore the land of Kingston Town, right outside of the Blue Mountains, that's mentioned in the lyrics. Meanwhile, I was down for the Blue Mountains north of Kingston based largely on my desire to emulate the Damian Marley song "Hey Girl," which features a line about "drinking Blue Mountain cappuccinos."

But now that I've chatted with all these Rastas, my initial love for the music has expanded into a deeper appreciation for Rastafari culture at large—especially in light of my role as a wellness editor. I've now come to regard Rastafarians as homegrown wellness mavens. Yet scientific backup on this idea is hard to find. While I'd love to be able to rattle off a bunch of solid statistics here about how Rastas who live from the earth, the Ital way, are XX percent healthier than Americans who feast on processed food, hardly any concrete research about the overall health and wellness of Rastafari exists. They just don't document that sort of stuff.

"Generally speaking, there's no catechism for this faith," cultural anthropologist Jake Homiak, PhD, a longtime Rastafari advocate who curated the *Discovering Rastafari!* exhibit at the Smithsonian's National Museum of Natural History, told me after my trip. In fact, like many alternative social movements that aren't supported by the dominant government, the history isn't documented in one place—so even that tends to vary a little bit depending on whom you ask. "That's the way it works in Rastafari, and that's the way it works in Jamaica: People are entitled to their own versions, and it's classified in multiple ways," he continued. Back at Stush in the Bush, Chris had also explained that Rastafarians don't really have any centralized marker at all. "There's no real Rastafari school. The ideologies and philosophies of Rastafari and Marcus Garvey are nowhere to be found in our political systems, even though they left such a legacy of things that could really reform the society. There's no real symbol of Rastafari society other than the music and the food and the culture," he explained. Ultimately, that means it's especially important for the world to recognize and honor those symbols.

There's a reggae song I loved when I was growing up called "Back to My Roots," by Steel Pulse, and after speaking with all of these Rastafari, I've realized that the secret to true, authentic well-being may have been in those song lyrics all along. True health comes from trying as best as we can to nourish our bodies and souls with fresh, simple, natural foods—*roots* foods—not the processed stuff that feeds Big Food rather than our souls.

It's important to remember that the Ital way of living is deeply rooted in oppression, and for me to acknowledge that I have not experienced that hardship myself. Still, the underlying message is loud and clear: Taking control of our health and wellness is not just a personal act but also a political one. It's about tying wellness to a greater sense of purpose—to be as self-reliant as possible—so that we don't have to support a society that's pushing the wrong messages. And that's a lesson that truly applies to everyone. "I believe that anyone in this world can choose to live an Ital lifestyle simply by becoming responsible for the doctoring of themselves," Jahlani told me as we were wrapping up our conversation. "In the end, Ital requires you to take ownership of your own wellness. It holds you responsible for understanding the politics of the world around you, and how it is that you wish to take those politics into yourself." Ital living is about the power many people have as conscious consumers to change the narrative. It may not change the *whole* narrative, which in many places is defined by systemic injustices that require complete overhauls. But it's a tangible start. And it starts from within.

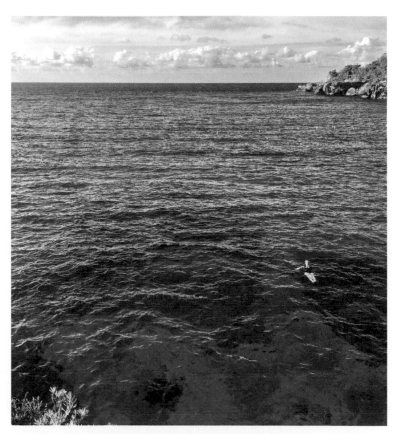

Negril: Spending time with Mother Nature is an
important part of the Ital lifestyle.

Live an Ital Life...

WHEREVER YOU ARE

Make your home your sanctuary.

As Chef Michael says, one of the easiest ways to resist commercialization is to create a "bubble of vibes" at home that makes you want to stay put. The key is to create your own personal refuge from society, whatever that means for you.

Connect to your food.

The best way to do this is to plant something. Being a seed parent, even if you're just watching a basil leaf grow on your windowsill, helps you feel more connected to nature overall. If planting something isn't an option, learn where your food comes from. Back at Stush in the Bush, Chris told me that he's often shocked to learn that people don't know how a carrot grows, even though they've eaten carrots their whole lives.

Look up at the sky each day.

Chronixx told me that he spends time outdoors each day not just for the fresh air but also for the reminder that we are all a small part of a much bigger natural universe. Rastafari believe that the more we acknowledge that connection, the more likely we are to feel grounded.

Go herbal.

Rastafari who strictly adhere to the rules of Ital are mostly booze-free, as too much alcohol decreases livity, and salt-free, as salt—at least the synthetic kind—is deeply tied to colonialism. Try swapping your next beer or glass of wine for herbal tea or herbal tonics or even fresh juice, and cooking with herbs and spices instead of salt. You'll likely get more health benefits, too.

Surround yourself with positive vibrations.

If you want to be inspired by messages of self-reliance and unity and hope in the face of oppression, listen to reggae! Chris told me that, like me, he throws it on when he needs a dose of Ital energy. "The music is a great way of getting the philosophies and the teachings without going anywhere," he said. "Just put on your headphones, and you'll be surrounded by positive vibrations, protected from the toxicity of the outside world."

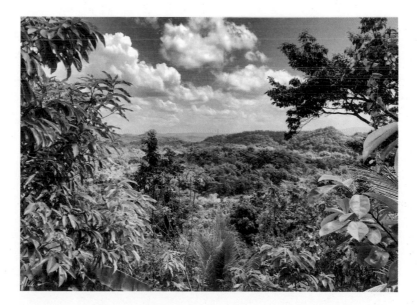

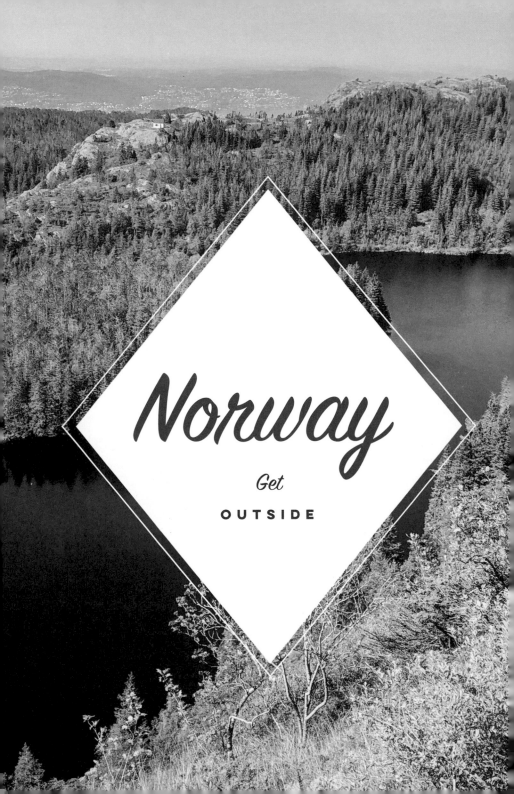

Norway

Get

OUTSIDE

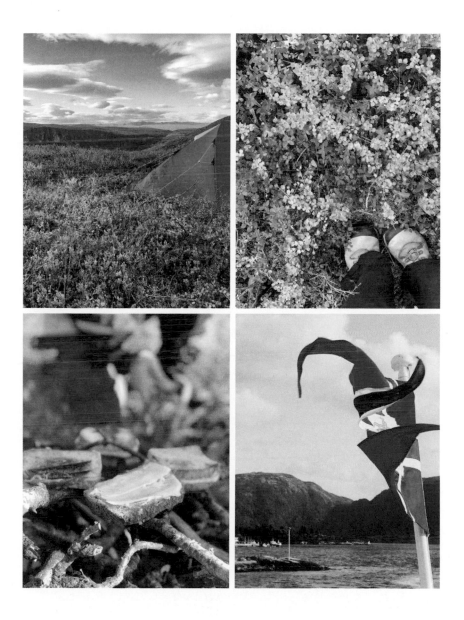

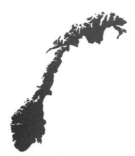

"HAVE YOU EVER hiked before?" my Norwegian trekking guide Barebra asked me with a sweet laugh. We were half an hour into my first hike in Norway, and I had already tripped over a patch of loose rocks, almost twisted my ankle, and fallen knee-deep into a hole of mud.

"Sort of a lot, actually," I replied sheepishly, thinking of the two-week trek I'd taken through the Andes Mountains in Peru, plus the countless day hikes I'd taken on my various other travels. I couldn't believe that the skills I'd gathered over the years weren't translating. On this trip, I was clearly the weakest link in my hiking group, the clumsy American caboose trying (and failing) to keep up with a crew of Norwegians in utter beast mode.

"It's so much harder here, though!" I laughed in an attempt to explain myself. "How is everyone else just flying up the mountain without tripping?"

"We've been hiking like this for our whole lives," Barebra replied. "Norwegian parents tend to bring their kids out for hikes as soon as they can walk, so the rocky terrain becomes second nature for all of us. We hardly even notice it because we've always hiked like this. It's the friluftsliv way."

I should've known. Like most travelers who have ever seen a single photo of Norway's stunning fjords—long, narrow, and deep inlets of sea between high cliffs—I'd wanted to visit them for as long as I can remember. But I'd actually come to Norway to investigate the very concept Barebra mentioned—friluftsliv—which I'd heard was completely entrenched in Norwegian society.

LOOSELY TRANSLATED, *FRILUFTSLIV* MEANS "THE FREE AIR LIFE."

My friend Andrea, who grew up in Norway and now lives in Brooklyn, originally introduced me to the philosophy over dinner one night. Although friluftsliv—pronounced *free-loofts-liv*—is technically a noun that describes the art of living an outdoor lifestyle, it's more of a *feeling*, she told me, a fundamental longing most Norwegians have to spend as much time outside as humanly possible. Never mind the fact that Norway gets tons of rain every year, or that the sun doesn't even rise for three *months* in certain parts of the country—Norwegians are still dedicated to the cause of getting outside no matter what. And that's largely because they know that they'll improve their physical and spiritual well-being in the process. "We just don't feel like our best selves until we've gotten a bit of a rosy glow in our cheeks after spending some time in fresh air," Andrea explained.

I'd left our dinner that night feeling enticed by that mindset, by the idea of having such unwavering devotion to the outdoors. I loved how spending time outside seemed like such a non-negotiable to many Norwegians and wondered if I could benefit from some of that spirit myself. I'd been feeling especially burnt out on urban New York City living at that point, and I knew that a large part of that was all the time I spent indoors. I've lived in the city for thirteen years now, and while I'm incredibly fortunate to get to travel a lot for my job, I still spend the majority of my waking hours indoors on my computer during the day, and then indoors again at night, either on the couch at home or at a bar or restaurant. Back when I worked on staff at the wellness magazine, I used to joke that I was like a little rat, scurrying underground on the subway from one indoor hideaway (my apartment in Brooklyn) to the other (my office in downtown Manhattan).

When I left my job to go out on my own as a freelancer, I thought I'd start spending much more time outside since I didn't need to have my butt in the chair at specific hours each day. And in some ways, I did: I was able to go on many more press trips (trips organized for journalists by tourism boards or hotels to promote their location or brand by introducing us to them firsthand) during the week than I had before. But when I was home in Brooklyn, my writing life turned out to be more of the same. If anything, it had actually become even easier to stay inside for the majority of the day if my presence wasn't required at a coffee meeting or a dinner date. I tried to go running most mornings or for an afternoon walk to guarantee that I would at least get out of the house for a nice chunk of time, but during the cold winter months, I often bailed on that plan and stayed inside in my sweatpants all day long.

According to the Environmental Protection Agency (EPA), I was definitely in the majority: Americans spend approximately 90 percent of their time indoors. That means we're spending only 10 percent of our time reaping the health benefits of Mother Nature, and the majority of our time breathing stale air inside, where the EPA says that the concentrations of some pollutants are two to five times higher than they are outside. And that's not exactly good for our health. Heavy indoor air pollutants can lead to headaches, dizziness, fatigue, respiratory diseases, heart disease, and cancer.

I'd been wanting to make the outdoors a much bigger part of my weekly routine, but to make matters worse, the indoor life was having a cultural moment. Brands were cashing in on the trend with sheet masks and fuzzy blankets that signified a new truth: *Staying in is the new going out*. At work, I got lots of proposals from brands who wanted to "align" their products with hygge, the Danish way of living that prioritizes coziness as the key to a happy life. Any Dane will tell you that you can't buy your way into hygge with fleece socks and a candle. But the overriding marketing message was that it's okay—trendy, even—to spend so much time indoors, especially when you have the products to make your stay more comfortable.

There were even new indoor workout classes that simulated the outdoors, like virtual runs and bike rides that transported you to tropical locales around the world. Back at the magazine, I sampled a boot camp class at "the world's first cold temperature gym" that charged people $34 to simultaneously freeze their asses off and get in shape. I'm all for the science behind cold-weather workouts—research has shown that you may burn more calories and can enhance your endurance—but doesn't, oh I don't know, just going outside do the same thing?

When I first heard about friluftsliv from Andrea, I immediately thought of a group of ski-town bros I went to college with, who now live in "rad" places like Tahoe and Boulder and say things like "gnarly run" and "crushing IPAs." Back in college, these guys lived for fresh powder and Patagonia everything, and spent all of their winter breaks out on the slopes. I wondered if a friluftsliv devotee would simply be Norway's version of the Tahoe bro or bro-ette. But it turns out, I was wrong.

FRILUFTSLIV ISN'T JUST AN ADVENTUROUS HOBBY— IT'S A STATE OF MIND. Children learn about friluftsliv in outdoor kindergartens (yes, outdoor!), and the country's universities even offer college degrees in the philosophy. Nearly every city in Norway has a chapter of the Norwegian Trekking Association, a government-run organization founded in 1868 whose job it is to promote friluftsliv and make the surrounding nature as accessible as possible so that everyone can participate. (Think of it like our National Parks Conservation Association, if we had a national park in nearly every city around the country.) Norway even has an intricate cabin system associated with friluftsliv, where Norwegians can stay in government-owned cabins scattered throughout the country, as long as they respect the property while they're there and leave money in the envelope by the door when they leave (it's a total honor system). The cabins are stocked with blankets and sheets, and some of them even have food, like dried soup mixes and premade campfire dinners.

The History of Friluftsliv

While the legal definition of friluftsliv *is "the amount of time you spend outside apart from organized sports," its cultural roots run far deeper. Here's how the term fits into Norwegian history:*

1814: Norway gained independence from Denmark and attempted to gain independence from Sweden. Norwegians were left trying to figure out what made them distinctively Norwegian, and realized that they were the only Scandinavians who had mountains— so the idea of the mountain-loving Norwegian was born.

1859: The term *friluftsliv* was originally coined by the famous Norwegian playwright and poet Henrik Ibsen at the beginning of the second wave of the Industrial Revolution. Ibsen was relaxing in a cottage in the woods, staring into the flames of a fire, and wrote, ". . . This is friluftsliv for my thoughts." At first, only the rich intellectual Norwegian aristocrats and artists like Ibsen could afford to go out and explore the mountains, as the working class was too busy mining and manufacturing in the textile mills. But, much like the Industrial Revolution in the US, the Industrial Revolution in Norway gave workers more rights, spare time, and money—so more people were able to go out into nature. Friluftsliv, then, became a status symbol, and soon enough, a national pastime and way to celebrate your Norwegian identity.

1957-PRESENT DAY: Norway instituted the Outdoor Recreation Act, which made it legal for Norwegians to roam freely across the country. This "right to roam"—called *allemansrätten*—guarantees that everyone has the right to experience nature. Today, allemansrätten also exists in Sweden. Norwegians and Swedes are both allowed to walk through and even camp on any piece of uncultivated land in the countryside, forests, or mountains, as long as they keep at least 500 feet away from the nearest inhabited house or cabin—and show respect for both the locals and the surrounding wilderness. (Those who want to stay in the same place for more than two nights must get permission from the landowner, too, unless they are deep in the wilderness.)

Even though friluftsliv is a point of Norwegian national pride, I still wondered: *Do* all *Norwegians celebrate nature all the time?* I'd heard that Norwegians love to tell you how there's no bad weather, only bad clothing—but is that really true across the board? Is this idea more concentrated in certain places? How often do most Norwegians get out into nature, really—don't they have office jobs, too? I knew our different infrastructures meant that Americans can't exactly set up camp on someone else's land like Norwegians do, and I also wasn't expecting to come home with magical skiing abilities or sculpted trail running abs. But I wanted to know if and how I and other Americans could live a more friluftsliv lifestyle in our day-to-day existence.

My plan was to start in Bergen, where Andrea grew up, as her mom had graciously offered to host me. Nicknamed Norway's "City of Seven Mountains," Bergen—the second-largest city in Norway after the capital Oslo—always seems to make its way to the top of those "best cities in Europe" lists, and for good reason. While Oslo is considered to be the most metropolitan, internationally focused city in Norway, known for its coffee culture and edgy architecture, Bergen is celebrated for its charming wooden houses, picturesque harbor, and mountainous landscapes. Andrea assured me that it was the perfect place to start my friluftsliv quest, as many locals there—including her mom—weave nature treks into their lives every single day.

Then, after I got my bearings in Bergen, I planned to head north. Way north. I'd stop in Sogndal, a university town about five hours north of Bergen that's home to one of the country's strongest friluftsliv departments, before heading even farther north to Alta, my final stop, where I was going to visit Alta Folkehogskole, a "folk high school" dedicated entirely to friluftsliv. (Alta Folkehogskole was formerly known as *Oytun*— pronounced *aye-tune*—which is what most people still call it.) Folk high schools are a particularly Scandinavian concept, popular in Norway, Sweden, Finland, and Denmark. They're meant for students age eighteen and up who have taken a gap year between high school and college, and are usually based around a single skill like writing or art or, in Oytun's case, friluftsliv. There are eighty folk high schools around Norway, and they're all tuition-free, though you do have to pay for room and board, trips, and supplies. They also don't do exams or grades, focusing instead on life lessons and making genuine connections. About 11 percent of Norwegian youth end up going to one of them before university to simply enjoy themselves and have a good time, as the lack of competition and focus on figuring out how you want to live your life make them the perfect breeding ground for lifelong friendships. Andrea's older sister Signy, who now lives outside Washington, DC, went to Oytun when she was eighteen. She told me I *had* to go when I was in Norway: "You can't write about friluftsliv without visiting Oytun, because it's the epicenter of the entire philosophy— Oytun *is* friluftsliv."

Starting in Bergen and making my way up to Oytun was an ambitious itinerary, no doubt. But I was hopeful that, after exploring both urban and remote lands, I'd have a better understanding of the extent to which friluftsliv exists around the country—and the ways we can weave those practices into our own lives at home.

WHEN I TOUCHED DOWN IN BERGEN, IT WAS SURPRISINGLY WARM AND UNCHARACTERISTICALLY SUNNY FOR A CITY KNOWN FOR ITS RAINFALL.

Andrea's mom, Ragnhild, was waiting at the airport with a sign that said "Annie." After we introduced ourselves with a hug (we'd never met, but we figured we were on hugging terms already), she brought me to the train to begin the journey to her apartment.

"One of the reasons that I love living here in Bergen is that I get up and go out and enjoy myself every single day," Ragnhild told me after I'd gotten my bags all situated on my lap on the train. She's lived in the city since the early 1990s, with no plans of leaving, ever—and as I watched quaint, thatched-roof houses and endless mountain backdrops pass us by in the window, I was already beginning to see why.

"Now that I'm retired," Ragnhild continued, "I wake up in the morning, make breakfast, and then pack a sandwich to take with me on my daily hike—Bergen is a great city for daily hikes." To be clear, her daily hike isn't always in the wilderness. Mostly, it's walking through town doing errands. But as a Norwegian, she told me, she was raised to believe that walking outside should be part of your daily routine no matter what.

"That sounds very friluftsliv to me," I remarked, hoping I'd actually pronounced it right.

Ragnhild laughed. "Friluftsliv doesn't really have a definition. It's more of a feeling, an urge to get outside because you don't feel like yourself if you stay indoors," she mused. But after she thought about it for a bit, she concluded that yes, her daily hikes were friluftsliv—she just hadn't defined it in that way before because she hadn't really defined it at all. "It's so ingrained in the way that Norwegians operate that it's almost beyond words," she continued. "It's how we live. I always go out during the day, because that's what I grew up doing." Most days, she walks to get bread from her favorite bakery, and the fish she likes from the fish market. And somewhere in between all that walking, she stops to eat her packed lunch so she can keep on walking after that. "Walk, walk, walk, and then walk some more—every Norwegian knows that."

I spent the next couple of days immersing myself in the Norwegian lifestyle, trying to mimic Ragnhild's ways. Andrea's sister Signy happened to be visiting Bergen with her two kids while I was there, and every morning, she and Ragnhild would put out a "typically Norwegian" full breakfast spread, including three different types of bread (whole-wheat sourdough, a dark brown bread loaded with seeds, and a plain white loaf), plus smoked salmon, hard-boiled eggs, freshly cut cucumber and tomato slices, yogurt, a package of salami, a huge hunk of cheese paired with a cheese slicer, and the infamous "brown cheese"—a distinctly Norwegian specialty made from goat's milk and whey. (People in Norway love to talk about their opinions about brown cheese. Like it or hate it, sharing your take on it is a big cultural unifier.)

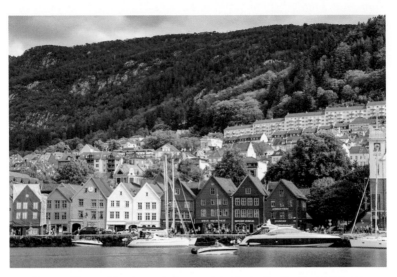

Bergen: No need to choose between charming waterfront row houses and fresh mountain trails.

After breakfast, Ragnhild would put out parchment paper so that we could pack sandwiches for our lunches later on. "We eat a *lot* of bread in Norway, probably more than in most other cultures," Ragnhild told me on my first morning. "But I think it's because our bread is so much better than it is in other places around the world." As a traveler who's eaten bread in a whole bunch of those other places, I agree. Norwegian bread is heavenly: much denser, grainier, and more flavorful than other kinds.

Most afternoons, I explored Bergen on my own, going for hikes and wandering into bars and coffee shops to see if anyone would want to chat friluftsliv with a random American. I fell in love with the city's built-in juxtaposition, how it's possible to walk out of a cute shop downtown, look up, and catch a view of Mount Fløyen, Bergen's most popular mountain of the seven.

And I especially loved Bryggen, Bergen's famous historic wharf district located on the east side of the harbor that was named a UNESCO World Heritage Site in 1979. I'd seen countless photos of its iconic side-by-side wooden row houses in travel magazines and on Instagram, with adjectives like "magical" and "dreamy" and "storybook" floating around in the hashtags, and I was happy to learn that the photos hadn't been enhanced— the classic postcard shot really was as picturesque as it appears. But it was the tiny alleyways *behind* the well-documented row houses that delighted me even more. Dotted with old creaky-floorboard gift shops and adorable window-box cottages, they were the kind that make you wonder what it would be like to move in, to *live* there, to wake up and get your morning coffee from that cute place on the corner.

As the days went by, I began to realize that, as Ragnhild said, the meaning of friluftsliv is indeed very loose—most Norwegians have developed their own personal definition. One coffee barista told me that, for her, friluftsliv is like a daily vitamin, one she has to have regularly. "Nature is a part of Norwegians, I think, much more than it is for other people," she told me as she prepared my latte. "We feel lost without getting our fill each day." Another local, a bartender originally from Norway's Lofoten Islands, told me that, to him, friluftsliv is a backpack, because it symbolizes freedom. "All you need to do is pack a sandwich and a thermos of coffee in your backpack, and go outside and just roam. That's happiness."

My favorite friluftsliv definition of all, though, came from one of my hiking guides, Cecile. We spent a full day together climbing up and around Mount Fløyen, admiring the stunning views of the fjords below. Cecile had brought us a packed lunch (pancakes, brown cheese sandwiches, and a thermos full of hot coffee), and we chose a gorgeous, windy spot near the top of the mountain to plop down and enjoy our meal. When I asked her to define friluftsliv as we were sitting there, her first reaction was to laugh. "You Americans, always trying to define Scandinavian words!" she joked. But then: "It's hard to pinpoint what it is, exactly. It's just this feeling that you get when you're out in nature and you look around and you take a deep breath and it's just . . . ahhh. Your brain sort of just shuts off, and you can finally relax." Sitting up there on the mountain with her, breathing in the crisp, fresh air with the occasional whiff of brown cheese, I started to understand what she meant. Perhaps friluftsliv is one great big giant exhale.

On my last day in Bergen, I had coffee with Sabine Koch, the marketing coordinator for the Bergen chapter of the Norwegian Trekking Association. As a German who moved to Bergen a decade ago, Sabine and her husband are now raising their kids there, and I thought she'd be a great person to talk to because she comes from an outside perspective but she works on the inside. I'd heard a lot of various friluftsliv definitions over the past few days and asked for her expert opinion on their common themes. "They all speak to the typically Norwegian feeling that friluftsliv is ultimately an urge you can't escape—Norwegians *need* to be outside," she explained, telling me she'd never seen anything like it back home in Germany. "Most of them are so connected to nature that they need it to make it through a single day. From early childhood, it's part of their whole lives." For many of them, I realized, it *is* their whole life.

How Nature Rx Can Help
You Feel Your Best

Environmental psychologists have been studying the strong link between spending time outside and well-being for decades, and in the past few years, doctors have even started to prescribe nature walks for their patients—a therapeutic technique known as ecopsychology. Here are a few key research-backed benefits to friluftsliv-ing:

DEEP RELAXATION: What Cecile describes as a "giant exhale" is likely based on the idea that she's not having to deal with responding to anything—what psychologists refer to as "bids" from the outside world. When there isn't a demand forcing you to pay attention, it's much easier to relax.

IMPROVED CREATIVITY: Without these "bids" from the outside world, your mind may also go one step further and start connecting loose ideas in ways it wouldn't have in more structured environments. But sooner or later, nature will present something that draws you back in—a bird chirping, a pretty tree. Researchers theorize that this ebb and flow between daydreaming and "effortless engagement," in which you enjoy the birdsong without having to think about it, ultimately boosts creativity.

BETTER CONCENTRATION: This "effortless engagement" with your surroundings also gives your brain a chance to rest and restore—an idea scientists call *attention restoration theory*. And like most things in life, allowing your concentration to take a break means you may be better able to pay attention later on.

STRENGTHENED EMPATHY: This one's like a chain reaction: The more time you spend in nature, the more likely you are to feel motivated to keep it clean and beautiful for years to come. And researchers have found that inspiration to be better can bubble over into other areas of your life, too.

A couple weeks before my trip to Norway, I'd emailed a Norwegian professor named Tom Lund, who teaches outdoor education and Nordic friluftsliv at the Western Norway University of Applied Sciences in Sogndal. I'd learned through my research that this particular university is known for their friluftsliv department, so I thought it would be fitting to spend some time there before making my way to the folk high school up in Alta. Located right on Norway's longest and deepest fjord, Sognefjord, Sogndal is much smaller and more remote than Bergen, with only 7,000 residents in comparison to Bergen's 272,000. From the school's website, I could see that Tom was one of the heads of the friluftsliv department and looked to be about my age, so I hoped he'd be open to my (admittedly random) request. I asked if he'd like to meet up for an interview or perhaps a hike, and to my delight, he invited me to join him in Sogndal for a "typically Norwegian pure friluftsliv weekend" with his friends, filled with long hikes, cooking food over a fire, and foraging for fungi. Obviously I was in!

I ARRIVED IN SOGNDAL FROM BERGEN LATE FRIDAY NIGHT AFTER A GORGEOUS FIVE-HOUR FERRY RIDE THROUGH THE FJORDS.

The next morning, Tom and his girlfriend, Marie, picked me up at my hotel to go on our first adventure, a hike along the fjord with two of their other friends. I'd only chatted with Tom on the phone at that point, but it felt comfortable from the moment we met in person—he and Marie treated me like a friend from the get-go. After I got in the car, we drove to the grocery store to buy a couple loaves of bread and tubed jalapeño cheese to eat for lunch in the mountains. "Tubed cheese is so convenient—it's one of our favorite hiking foods," Tom assured me as we were shopping. "All you need to do is squeeze it out onto some bread when you're hungry, and it'll fill you up and give you energy for more hiking."

Standing there in the dairy aisle of the grocery store, contemplating how many tubed cheeses to buy, I started thinking about Norwegians' relationship to food. I'd eaten some version of bread and cheese on every hike back in Bergen, too. And although I hadn't eaten at any five-star restaurants yet, from my experience living the local life, I took it that Norwegians equate food with sustenance: something that will help them stay outside for longer without letting hunger drag them down. I thought of all of the wellness food options back in New York, from "wellness shots" to $14 grain bowls to $9 green juices, and realized I hadn't even seen the word *wellness* in Norwegian grocery stores at all so far. I'd seen nourishing items on their own—lots of fresh seafood, fruits and vegetables, and boatloads of grainy bread and cheese, to name a few—but the actual word *wellness*? Nope.

Of course, I knew that it would be impossible to go back home and say, "Well, that does it—I will abandon all 'wellness' foods and live on bread and cheese for the rest of time." Nutrition doesn't work like that, and the Norwegians I spoke with may simply be built differently. But still, on a more philosophical level, their utilitarian approach to food did make me wonder: Did I think about healthy food too much? It's no secret that many Americans are obsessed with this topic. But even though there's a proven link between healthy food and overall well-being, many Americans make that connection without even thinking about the actual science. Meanwhile, most of the

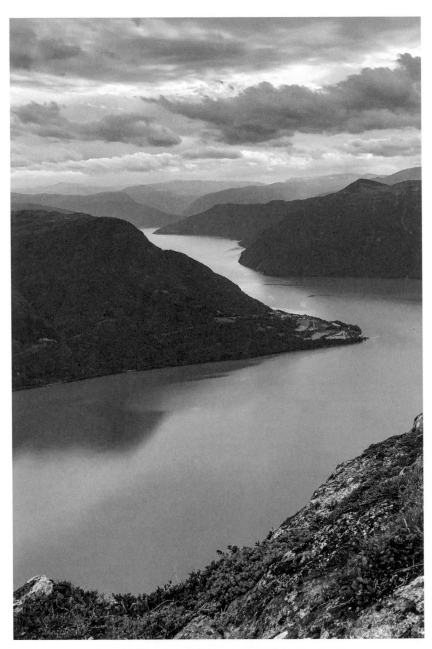

Sogndal: The view of the aqua fjords from the top of
the mountain was worth the grueling climb.

Norwegians I spoke with did no such thing, instead seeking out their wellness from the great outdoors. Rather than glorifying food the way we often do here, they saw it as sustenance, plain and simple. To them, the hike was always about the hike, not about packing the perfect lunch for the hike. The sandwiches were simply part of the hike.

When we got to the trailhead, two of Tom's other friends, Stian and Helle, were waiting for us in the parking lot. Like Tom and Marie, they smiled and welcomed me into the group right away, immediately making me feel at home. But they also looked super fit, decked out in bright blue activewear, and I started to worry that I wouldn't be able to keep up. Turns out, I wasn't all that wrong. Like my first stumbling and fumbling hike in Bergen, this one was also incredibly steep, complete with loose rocks and sticks and, the closer we got to the top, puddles of mud. "You guys can go ahead if you want," I told the crew as I inched my way forward. "I'm definitely not used to these hills!"

Marie, Stian, and Helle continued on, but Tom stayed behind with me, probably to make sure I didn't die. "You know, most Norwegians are really fast hikers because we grew up hiking from such a young age—but friluftsliv isn't actually about speed at all," he told me. **"I TEACH MY STUDENTS THAT IT'S ABOUT SLOW-ING DOWN AND GETTING IN TUNE WITH YOURSELF AND WITH YOUR SURROUNDINGS.** It doesn't matter how long it takes you to get up the mountain, as long as you feel yourself connecting to the nature."

I immediately felt more at ease once Tom reminded me to focus on how my brain felt rather than my legs. But sadly, that cerebral mindset is becoming slightly less common these days.

"I'm worried about the future of friluftsliv, to be honest," Tom told me as we continued to trudge on up the mountain. As a well-respected professor of friluftsliv, he's read nearly all of the literature on the philosophy out there, and now he's on a mission to preserve the concept in its truest, most authentic form. "I know that you're writing about getting away from the commercialization of wellness, but friluftsliv has started to get commercialized recently, too," he said. Brands have started marketing all of the latest outdoor gear and clothing as friluftsliv style, he told me, and younger Norwegians—especially those who grew up with social media—are beginning to think that friluftsliv can only be achieved if you're wearing the latest fleece. "Many of my young students come into my class thinking that they need to own the best new hiking poles, and the most expensive down jacket since they're taking a friluftsliv class. They see this stuff on Instagram and think that they need it, too," Tom continued. But his whole goal as a professor is to bring them outside into the mountains to show them the original pre–social media meaning of the term. "I'm trying to help them realize that it's a bodily and spiritual experience . . . that it's all about disconnecting from the noise and reconnecting with nature and with themselves."

Of course, we all know that disconnecting from the noise is getting harder and harder when the noise is getting louder and louder. And that's truer than ever in Norway. With 5.7 million overnight visitors in 2018, Norway is struggling with major overtourism these days, thanks in large part to Trolltunga, one of its outstanding hiking spots with a killer—and very Instagrammable—view that exploded on social media. You've probably seen the shot: It's the one where some tourist or travel influencer is standing on what looks like a super-high diving board made of stone and could, in theory, get knocked over by the wind and plummet to their death into the fjord below. That potential drama is what makes the photo so epic, of course, and it's why many people go on the grueling 15-mile hike to get there in the first place. In 2018, Trolltunga had ninety thousand visitors, up from only one thousand visitors just a decade ago. But Tom is very concerned about the impact this influx will have on Norway's friluftsliv spirit in the years to come: "To me, friluftsliv is about getting deep into nature, and using that time

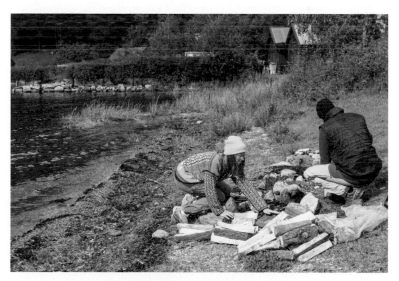

Sogndal: Tom's friends all know that making a
fire outside is a friluftsliv essential.

with no one around to decompress. But now it's getting harder to find those spots."

The next morning, Tom and Marie picked me up at my hotel again to head out to the mountains. Tom had organized a post-hike dinner the night before with a couple of his other friends, too, and I was feeling so grateful that they'd all welcomed me into their group so openly. We cooked steak and roasted vegetables, drank wine, and played card games, and as the night was winding down, Tom's friend Ingelin started telling everyone about how she'd shot her first reindeer the other day (classic Norway). It was currently sitting in her freezer.

"Shall we have a reindeer cookout in the mountains tomorrow?" she asked the group. The answer was a resounding yes, so a plan was hatched: We'd meet at a lake in the mountains, make a fire, and cook Ingelin's conquest over the flames. My first Sunday in Sogndal would be Reindeer Day.

Norwegians have a special relationship with Sundays. Back in New York, Andrea had told me that she grew up going hiking every Sunday, and most Norwegians I'd met, including my new Sogndal friends, said the same. The tradition goes back to the Industrial Revolution, when workers were first getting rights to experience the wonder of friluftsliv. Because they didn't have as much money as the aristocrats and still had to work, they couldn't spend as many consecutive days in the mountains— so they started taking mini excursions on Sundays to whatever nature was close by. The tradition stuck, and Nature Sundays continue to be an integral part of Norwegian culture.

By the time we reached the lake, it was around 2 p.m., and Stian and Helle and a few others were building the fire to start cooking. (Thanks to the right to roam, Norwegians are able to make a fire anywhere they want, as long as they respect the nature around them.) The reindeer tasted fairly mild and much less gamey than I thought it would, and after we ate, we all sat around drinking coffee and staring at the fire. Pretty soon, it started to rain, and I was all set to pack it up and transfer the rest of the reindeer picnic to someone's apartment when I looked around and realized that everyone had already put on their rain gear instead. I hadn't even noticed their lightning-fast response.

"Don't you want to put on your raincoat?" Marie asked me when she saw me getting wet.

"I do, I just wasn't as quick to get mine out!"

"I guess we're pretty used to it," she laughed.

We spent the rest of the afternoon hanging around the lake in our raincoats and rain pants, lounging on fluorescent yellow foam camping mats that a few members of the group had brought, not the least bit concerned that it was wet out. It stopped raining after a while, but the grass was still damp and it was a bit chilly. I've gotta say, if I were on my own, I definitely would've called it quits and gone home to read or watch TV. At one point, as I was lying there on one of the foam mats, I thought, "Seriously, do Norwegians *ever* want to go inside?"

BY THE TIME I MADE IT UP TO OYTUN, THE FOLK HIGH SCHOOL IN ALTA AND MY FINAL AND NORTHERNMOST STOP ON MY NORWAY JOURNEY, I WAS SICK.

I woke up in my hotel room in Sogndal the morning after the rainy reindeer cookout with a stuffy nose and a throbbing headache, proof that my fairly indoors-y body wasn't handling so much consecutive friluftsliv-ing all that well. And the flight to Alta made it even worse. My ears started ringing in pain, and I had to ask the flight attendant for medicine. The Croatian man sitting next to me was very concerned that I was traveling alone and was so under the weather. "I hope you'll get the chance to rest when you get to Alta," he told me.

"Rest?" I laughed and shook my head. "Far from it." Oytun offers classes on things like nature photography, kayaking, rock climbing, hunting and fishing, backcountry skiing, and even Arctic dog sledding. And after emailing with Oytun's headmaster, Henning Iversen, we'd decided I would go on a two-day camping excursion with the nature photography class, with the hopes of documenting the Northern Lights. "I'm going camping in the wilderness for a couple of days," I told my new Croatian friend. "I'll be sleeping under the stars in freezing-cold temperatures."

He shook his head in sympathy. Of all the times to get sick, the day before camping in Alta was not an ideal one. Alta is an extreme destination, the kind that gets a reaction when you tell people you're going there. Even people in Sogndal were impressed: "Oh wow, you're going all the way to *Alta*? That's so far." At 70 degrees north, it would be the farthest north I'd ever been. (New York City is 41 degrees north, for context; Reykjavik, Iceland, is 64.) And although peak Northern Lights–viewing season runs from October through March in Norway, it's still possible to see them as early as August—and I really hoped Alta would pull through with some colors.

When I woke up on my first morning in Oytun, my cold had miraculously improved overnight. I'd arrived in the dark late the night before, so I hadn't really gotten the chance to look around yet, and I was struck by the astonishing level of natural beauty that morning. The sky was a clear, bright blue, and I could see mountains in the distance, stretching on for miles and miles. My cabin overlooked a patch of tall pine trees, and it felt like a mix between summer camp and an L.L. Bean catalog, with two twin beds, red-and-blue plaid blankets, and smooth, paneled cedar walls that made the whole room feel even warmer than it was.

I made my way into the dining hall for the daily 7 a.m. breakfast, and all I could smell was toast. The bright morning light was streaming through tall glass windows, landing right on a student who was stacking at least ten slices of bread on top of each other into a very tall pile. Then I looked around, and it was more of the same: Norwegians everywhere, in gorgeous, bulky wool sweaters, sitting around cozy, candlelit wooden tables, smiling and stacking bread like Legos. Even Ragnhild, my Norwegian bread whisperer, hadn't prepared me for this level of loaves.

"Because we're going camping for four days straight, we need as many sandwiches as we can fit in our backpacks," one girl explained after I sat down next to her at her table. She was holding a big plastic Tupperware container filled to the brim with bread and cheese and salami sandwiches, and when I told her I was going camping for two days, she handed me a big hunk of parchment paper. "You're going to need this," she said. "If I were you, I'd make at least ten sandwiches."

And so it went at Oytun. If America runs on Dunkin', Oytun—and Norway in general—runs on bread. When I went to meet my group outside, the teacher, Per-Arne, immediately inquired about my food supply: "Did you make enough sandwiches?" This was clearly very important. I nodded yes and he said, "Good. That's a big part of what we do out there. Now hop in the van." I sat in the front seat between Per-Arne and a Swede named Max, with twelve eighteen-year-old Norwegians behind us (Max was the only non-Norwegian in the group). I knew I'd be sharing a tent with some of them later, which I felt a little weird about because I'd just met them, but I tried to let that thought go—and hoped they wouldn't mind my lingering sniffles.

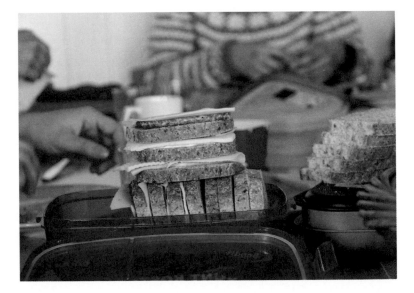

Alta: Norwegians do not mess around when it comes to packing sandwiches.

We spent the morning and early afternoon alternating between hiking, eating, and taking nature photos. Unlike Bergen and Sogndal, the terrain in Alta was flat and squishy, not steep and rocky, which helped me keep my balance while wearing such a heavy backpack. Although I go camping quite often during the summer, I usually go car camping in the Catskills in New York, which, let's be real, is the outdoorsy equivalent of training wheels. It's *much* easier than remote backcountry camping, which requires you to carry all of your supplies on foot, sleeping bag and all, for hours on end—I wasn't used to such manual labor in pursuit of relaxation! By the time we reached our final camping destination, it was around 3 p.m., and I was exhausted. But I was also ecstatic. With no cell service to speak of, we were out there, man. And as anyone who has ever spent time in deep nature will tell you, there is an exhilarating sense of freedom that comes from being away from it all, from being unable to participate in society even if asked. People pay for digital-detox escapes now, where hotel staff members will quite literally hold your phone hostage for however long you pay them to, but I've always found those quite puzzling— why not just go somewhere where Mother Earth does the work for you?

We set up our three tents in a valley nestled between two mountains dotted with wildflowers, and there wasn't another soul in sight for miles and miles. It was just us, the mountains, and the wide open sky. Since the sun wasn't going to set until 9 p.m., though, I figured Per-Arne had some other activity planned for us, something we'd do to pass the time until we started looking for the Northern Lights. But nope. Max and some of the others got a fire going, and then, for the next few hours, we just . . . sat. There was occasional chatter, but not much. It was mostly deep fresh-air sighs.

At one point, around 7 p.m. or so, someone decided it was dinnertime, so everyone took their cold cheese sandwiches out of their Tupperware and held them over the fire on sticks, toasting them until they got crispy. Per-Arne had also brought a Ziploc bag of hot dogs and packaged tortillas to round out the meal. No one talked all that much during this cooking process, except to mutter the occasional "yessss" if they toasted their sandwich to utter perfection. And soon enough, it was back to sitting quietly. Even though we were a group of fifteen people, the only recurring sound was the crackling of the fire and the occasional rustle of the wind. I mastered what I came to call the "Norwegian sprawl," which is when you lie on your side with your head in one hand and just stare into the flames.

Sitting there watching the embers burn, I thought of all of the times I'd spent car camping with my American friends, when we busied ourselves with card games and set up fairly elaborate rigs, complete with chairs, coolers, cocktail mixers, and speakers for our tunes. Out in Alta, we didn't have those extras. And Per-Arne had a rule: No music in nature. Music disrupts friluftsliv, he told us, because we should be connecting with the sounds of Mother Earth.

As a huge music head, I didn't fully agree with him on that one, because listening to music helps me relax. But he did have a point. If I'd had it my way, I likely would've been playing campfire DJ, throwing on Tom Petty's "Wildflowers" to honor the surrounding wildflowers, or Neil Young's "Pocahontas," which

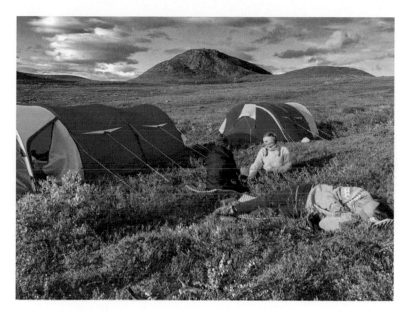
Alta: Could there be a prettier location for a Norwegian sprawl?

mentions the aurora borealis. But in the past few hours, I'd spent more time doing nothing and thinking about nothing than I had in a long while. As a freelance writer, I have a very busy mind, with a general low-grade sense of worry that pulses through it at all times: *Am I doing enough? What can I do better? Do I need to get more work? How can I make more money next month? Is this lifestyle sustainable over time? If it's not, what can I do to make sure that it is?* Though many of my worries turn out to be unfounded, the point is that they're there. But then, for the first time in a long time, they weren't. I was completely and utterly unplugged, disconnected from all technology and the rest of society, the farthest north I'd ever been, with no Wi-Fi to speak of and nothing to do but sit. While I spent the first hour or so thinking about practical things, like how I was going to organize my notes for this book and if my photos captured the spirit of Norway and did I have a clean hoodie for the hike home, my mind eventually drifted off into the abyss.

I don't know how long I zoned out for, or what broke me out of my reverie, exactly, but at one point my brain came back and it hit me: *This* is what we're missing. We've gotten so disconnected from nature that we've lost the ability to just be—and Mother Earth can help us reconnect with that fundamental part of ourselves. I felt deeply relaxed in a core sort of way, not because I'd gone to a yoga class but because I'd actually unplugged. Thanks in part to our lack of cell service, and in part to Per-Arne's insistence that we listen to the sounds of nature, I'd taken the opportunity to stare into the flames and chill. And the mental clarity that followed confirmed what the friluftsliv devotees had been telling me all along: Nature is the best medicine.

We were all in some version of the Norwegian sprawl when the cold began to take hold. It was around 8 p.m., just as the sun was beginning to set, and I booked it to the tent to fetch my two merino-wool base layers and my second down jacket. But once I had on all the layers I'd brought, including my raincoat and rain pants to block the wind, I still couldn't get warm.

I was envious of all the Norwegians who'd brought their thick Norwegian wool sweaters, and wished I had one of my own. "These wool sweaters are the only thing that will keep you warm out here," one of the girls told me with a sympathetic smile. I got so cold that I had to go curl up in my sleeping bag in the tent while we waited for the Northern Lights, and I wasn't

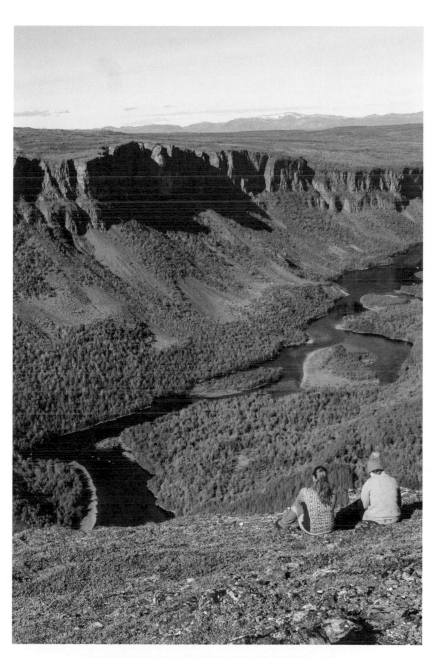

Aurland: Admiring the view over Aurlandsdalen Valley,
often referred to as Norway's Grand Canyon.

even sure I'd be able to make it out of there to witness the potential magic at all.

Finally, around 11 p.m., Per-Arne let us know: They were here. The lights. We'd lucked out, and the sky was delivering. Though they weren't visible to the naked eye, he could see them through his camera, trippy and green as ever, and it was time to shoot. I willed myself out of my sleeping bag, and set up my tripod with the others.

The photos themselves turned out pretty crappy, but I'm surprisingly okay joining Team Travel Memory on this one. The experience really was enough, one of those moments where it was just, *wow*, how do I actually live here on this Earth? In the past couple years, researchers have begun to study this sense of awe, and have found that it can help you feel lighter in spirit, more generous to other people, and more satisfied with your life. It can even make you feel as though you have more time to simply exist, all because the perspective shift helps put your worries in context. I co-sign that. Despite the frigid temperatures, I felt so limitless in that moment, so free and open and receptive to new thoughts. While I was standing there, watching the green glow appear like magic through my lens, I realized that Mother Nature had come through with an especially timely message: Just because you can't see it doesn't mean it's not there. It was the ultimate reminder that there's a deeper world lurking just beneath the surface if you make enough time to find it.

The next morning, I woke up before the others and unzipped the tent ever so quietly to take a walk to the bathroom (aka a clump of trees). The grass was wet with dew and a little bit crunchy from the cold, so I was careful to tiptoe away from our campsite so as not to wake the others with my shuffling. When I got back to the tent, I plopped my rain jacket down on a sunny patch of grass nearby, lay down on my back, took a deep breath à la Cecile in Bergen, and stared up at the sky to continue processing the Northern Lights events from the night before. Everyone I met in Norway had told me that friluftsliv was hard to define, that it's slightly different for everyone, that finding your own definition is a personal journey—and I knew in that moment that I'd finally found mine. It's about honoring Mother Nature's ability to guide us through our days. She is constantly dishing out lessons, even when we are too trapped in our indoor lives to really hear them.

Many of the Norwegians I met seemed to understand this take intuitively, a result of growing up with so much accessible nature all around. And after spending two weeks almost exclusively outside, I finally got it, too: Friluftsliv is making a point to hang out with Mother Nature whenever and wherever and as often as we can, so we can actually hear what she has to say.

Capture the Friluftsliv Spirit...

WHEREVER YOU ARE

Make every day an adventure.

Instead of dreading all of the items on your to-do list, try turning them into a daily hike like Ragnhild. If possible, run your errands on foot. If you'll be out for a while, bring a backpack and a sandwich.

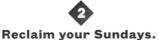

Reclaim your Sundays.

The concept of Sunday as an outdoor day has deep roots in Norwegian cultural history. The key is to label Sunday as your nature day in advance, so that you plan ahead. Americans may not have the "right to roam" on *all* land like Norwegians do, but you can invite friends and family to go on a hike or have a picnic.

Simplify your meals.

Food should be delicious and comforting, but not *every* meal has to be a production. Sometimes it can just feed you, or push you farther up the mountain. May I suggest a simple grilled cheese to start?

Embrace cold and rainy weather.

Most of us living with seasonal weather grumble about long winters and drizzly days, but Norwegians love the cold—and hardly mind the rain. Instead of hating on winter, think of the activities you can enjoy—like sitting by a crackling fire and going for walks through the snow. Invest in proper gear (rain pants are a must) and bust it out when the weather gets rough.

Seek out moments of awe.

Even if you are not surrounded by stunning, jaw-dropping scenery every day, it's still possible to experience the positive benefits of wonder—researchers say that the crucial element is a sense of vastness. Try watching awe-inspiring videos (the BBC's *Planet Earth* is always a good choice), reading inspiring stories of people doing incredible things like surfing 80-foot waves, or simply spending time with children—everything is new and vast for them.

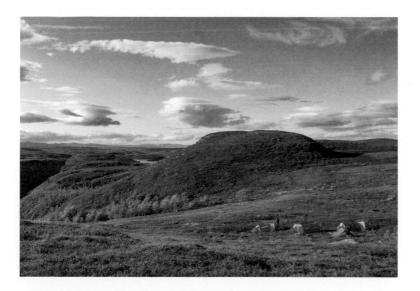

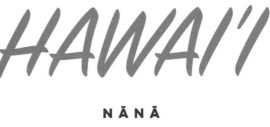

HAWAI'I

NĀNĀ

I KE KUMU

(Look to the Source)

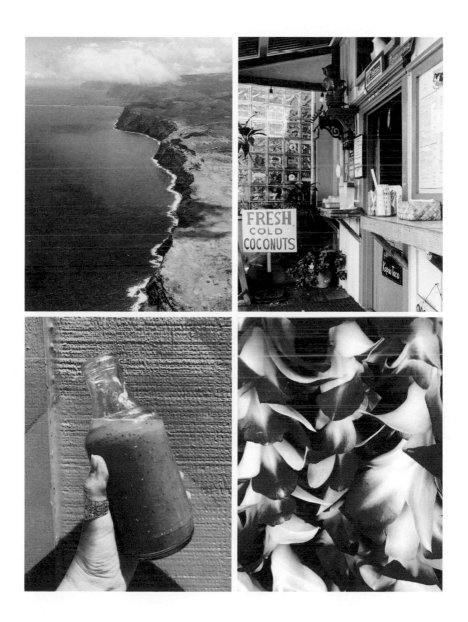

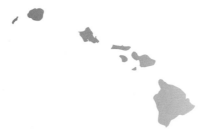

"**I** N ORDER TO live a healthy life in this world, you have to know your story."

Greg Solatario, a Native Hawaiian who lives on the same land where he grew up, told me this matter-of-factly one muggy afternoon in April. We had just finished a sweaty hike to a towering waterfall on his family's remote property on Molokaʻi, Hawaiʻi's fifth-largest island and arguably the sleepiest of the main six that tourists can visit. (Maui, Oʻahu, Kauaʻi, Lanai, and the island of Hawaiʻi—also known as the Big Island—are the other five.)

"I come from this land—my *family* comes from this land," he emphasized as he gestured to the surrounding tropical rain forest. "And I believe in a deep, deep way that knowing where I come from helps me stay healthy every day."

As a fiftieth-generation Solatario, Greg is part of the last ancient family still living in Halawa Valley, a historic piece of land on Molokaʻi where ancient Hawaiians settled as early as 650 CE. Theirs was the first functional village in all of the Hawaiian Islands, before it got wiped out by a famously devastating tsunami in 1946 and replaced by a thicket of hāpuʻu tree ferns and tropical fruit trees, like kukui, papaya, and mango. Today, the Solatarios live in an off-grid jungle house tucked among those very trees.

"There's a Hawaiian phrase, 'nānā i ke kumu,' which means 'look to the source,' or 'look to the teacher,'" he continued. The idea is that your ancestors are your guides, and you can look to them for all of the life wisdom you need. "When you know where you come from, you are better able to know yourself. And knowing yourself, knowing your own story, is one of the best ways to be well."

With a grand total of zero traffic lights, 7,345 permanent residents, and no nightlife to speak of, Molokaʻi isn't exactly a bumpin' destination—and that's a huge part of the allure for the ever-growing off-the-beaten-path crowd. There are miles of wild, untamed beaches—including one of Hawaiʻi's longest—plus rugged mountains, dramatic sea cliffs, and picturesque roads so empty, you can drive around belting out embarrassing pop songs with your windows down and no one will ever know. But sitting there watching that waterfall with Greg, listening to him share all sorts of wisdom about the art of living and the state of the world, I realized that the island's rural beauty was only part of the allure. The real allure was the Hawaiian spirit itself. I loved how the message of nānā i ke kumu was so focused on the past, when wellness—especially on the mainland—had begun to feel far too future-oriented for my liking. "This product will change your life" and other messaging implies that the answer has yet to be discovered. But nānā i ke kumu teaches us that the answer is already here. We don't need to buy our way into future wellness because we already have everything we need.

I've always known that Hawaiians have a special relationship to health and well-being. Growing up, I was fortunate enough to travel to the Big Island multiple times with extended family on my mom's side (there were just over twenty of us back then). My grandmother Betty, who died when I was in eighth grade, was especially obsessed with Hawaiian culture, which she claimed was the closest thing to her own personal religion. Hawaiians are connected to water in a deep way— many live by the phrase "ola i ka wai," which means "to get life from water"—and as a born-and-raised Southern California girl, Betty felt viscerally tied to the ocean, too. She was an incredible body surfer, and she was all about "communing with nature," both land and sea, to relieve stress and feel at peace in the world. My mom always says that Betty had "salt water in her veins," because, like many Hawaiians, she was bound to the waves. When Betty died, we scattered her ashes in the Pacific Ocean, and I still feel her presence whenever I'm swimming.

Those early Hawai'i trips could get a bit wild, with eleven young cousins just a few years apart. But Betty had her rules, and one of them was insisting that the grandkids spend some quiet time contemplating nature and communing with the Hawaiian sun gods each day. With the trade winds blowing softly in the afternoon, she'd gather us to make leis and shell necklaces, and we'd peacefully string the plumeria flowers or the shells one by one until one of the cousins started tugging at her sleeve or begging for another swim—and the spell would be broken. But for a few fleeting moments, I remember feeling something magical.

That's why I wanted to come back to Hawai'i as an adult to report on the wellness philosophies deeply embedded in Hawaiian culture. As I got older, the closest I got to Hawai'i was attending the occasional Polynesian-themed party, filled with plastic leis and aloha tiki mugs, and chatting with friends and coworkers who dreamed of leaving their mainland lives behind and heading to the islands. The word *aloha* these days has been misappropriated by people all over the world, becoming synonymous with escapism, or at least with the promise of paradise. And that's probably why, when most people think of wellness in Hawai'i these days, they think of the content Instagram dreams are made of: vibrant fruit smoothies, sunset surf sessions, yoga under palm trees, and anything else that reflects that "beach hair, don't care" lifestyle.

But I always knew that the true aloha spirit goes far deeper than visions of cocktail umbrellas. That tropical-screensaver imagery did not jibe with my own early, peaceful experiences on the Big Island, or with Betty's deep appreciation for Hawai'i's cultural and spiritual richness. So I asked the state's visitors bureau to help me get in touch with local Hawaiians across all of the islands who could help me further understand the true meaning behind the aloha spirit—and the wellness lessons embedded within its core philosophy. Greg was one of them, and I also met many others.

Without my cousins and on my own, I was able to explore all of the islands, and I fell for them even harder than I had as

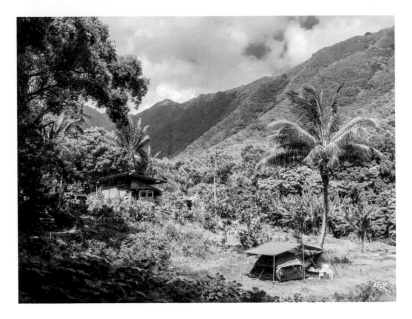

Moloka'i: Greg's family house tucked into the hapu'u tree ferns.

a kid. Yes, I ate ahi tuna poke bowls and fresh pineapple by day and watched gorgeous tropical sunsets by night, the kind that make you question your life choices and wonder what it would be like to witness that magenta sky on the regular. But the real magic happened when I met up with inspiring people on each island to "talk story," the local term for having a conversation.

During these chats, many Hawaiians shared their mo'olelo (the Hawaiian word for story, legend, or tradition) with me. They were quick to tell me that the meaning of aloha goes far deeper than hello and goodbye—it's about connection. And love. *"Alo* means to be face-to-face in one's presence, and *ha* means both the breath of life that we all share, and also humility," Uilani

Bobbit, a Hawaiian-language professor and lecturer at the University of Hawaiʻi at Mānoa, told me at one point during my trip. "So really, the spirit of aloha is about having true respect for everything around us, humans and the earth and ourselves, because we are all sharing the same air."

What I took away from our discussions most of all, though, even more than the actual definition of aloha itself, is that Hawaiians *looooove* to talk story, to share their moʻolelo. In some of the other countries I visited for this book, I often did other activities while interviewing my subjects, like going for a hike or cooking a meal together. But in Hawaiʻi, I mostly just . . . chatted. I sat, and I chatted. A woman I spoke with on Oʻahu told me that one of her favorite things about Hawaiʻi is that you can wear its scent on your skin, and I agree: The warm, soft air on all of the islands is an intoxicating mix of plumeria, jasmine, coconut, and salt, and it stuck on me like a heady all-day fragrance. But I would also add that the lessons I learned while talking story stuck with me long after the sweet scent faded away.

AND THE BIGGEST TAKEAWAY OF ALL? TALKING STORY *IS* THE STORY.

Whenever people ask me about my time in Hawaiʻi, I tend to skip over the glamour of Maui and the hippie shops of Kauaʻi and the black sand beaches of the Big Island and go straight to the conversations. I eventually get to the emerald-green mountains, and the lava deserts, and the poke, and the poi (a traditional Hawaiian dish made from the stem of the taro plant), but to me, the true beauty of Hawaiʻi lies in the art of communication itself. Hawaiian culture is rooted in oral storytelling. I could listen to Hawaiians talk all day—and I did. They tend to pull you in with their lyrical cadences and their rhythms and their ability to just *go* there, to the deep stuff, right away. Most Hawaiians, or at least the ones I spoke with, are incredibly skilled weavers of tales, which makes sense: The Hawaiian language itself was purely oral until the European missionaries came to the islands and formalized the alphabet in 1826 (more on that history in the box on page 94). They've been passing down stories for *generations*. And it's nearly impossible to talk about Hawaiian well-being without honoring this foundation first.

"Talking story is considered an important activity in Hawai'i because it was once a necessity: Hawaiian elders *had* to pass down their knowledge in order to keep it alive," Scott Saft, PhD, coordinator of the Hawaiian and Indigenous Language and Culture Revitalization program at the University of Hawaii at Hilo, told me. "And today, even though some of this information is now written down, it's still a way to continue that connectivity between generations—which is what well-being in Hawai'i is all about."

Even as a reporter, I felt connected to the people I talked story with just by listening to them speak. Psychologist Dr. Anne YJ Hsu, PhD, who specializes in identity issues and transcultural orientation, told me later over the phone why this made perfect sense. "When your relationship with someone is founded on storytelling time, that's how you connect and find meaning in your life," she began. To explain this concept further, she pointed to the difference between telling your own stories and reading someone else's story out loud. "When you're reading other people's stories, those stories are always in the third person. But when we're passing down oral stories—whether that's family stories, hometown stories, or even regional stories—the subjects are always 'I' or 'my' or 'your.' It's so much more relational when you say 'your great-grandfather said this,' or 'my neighbor said that.' There's a deeper connection there," she explained. "Listening to personal stories means you have been invited into a world of wonder by someone you love who's older and wiser and stronger and protects you, and that interaction is really powerful. It can foster a deep sense of well-being."

Hearing Dr. Hsu's explanation crystalized another truth I'd picked up on during my travels: Hawaiians *know* stuff about Hawai'i. It's not often that I meet someone in New York who regularly drops historical references about the city into casual conversation, but in Hawai'i? That's standard practice. Part of that is due to sheer geography. Just look at a map: The islands

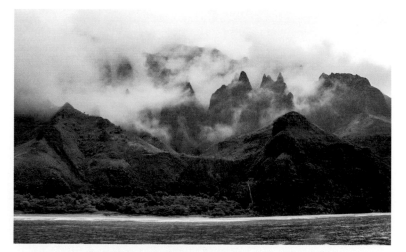

Kaua'i: Hawaiian mythology includes legends and stories about the Na Pali Coast's rugged sea cliffs.

are quite literally the most isolated landmass on Earth, farthest away from any sort of mainland than any other island in the world. With that in mind, it makes sense that Hawaiians know their history. Their isolation has created a close-knit community by the law of unintended consequences.

But it's bigger than that, too. Hawaiians also know their history because they're *proud* of their history. They're in awe of their ancestors. And why wouldn't they be? Native Hawaiians have lived on the islands since the Polynesians sailed there and proceeded to settle there in the fifth century CE. Up until the British explorer Captain James Cook arrived in 1778, it was just them and Mother Earth.

"THE SECRET TO OUR ANCESTORS' SURVIVAL WAS A CONCEPT KNOWN AS *ALOHA 'ĀINA,* WHICH TRANSLATES TO 'LOVE OF THE LAND,'" Anela Evans, a Hawaiian cultural practitioner based in Lanai, explained to me one sunny afternoon as we cruised around the dusty island in her jeep.

I'd taken the forty-five-minute ferry ride over from Maui earlier that morning (it's the only way to get to Lanai), and I was already enamored by the island's steep sea cliffs and its barren and seclusive feel. With a population of just around 3,000 people, in comparison to denser O'ahu's 953,000, parts of the island feel like another, far-less-crowded planet, with Mars-like rock gardens stretching on for miles and miles. "In ancient Hawaiian culture, every living thing in nature, from plants to animals to trees, had a deity attached to it. And our ancestors worshipped those deities every day," Anela, who earned her master's degree in Hawaiian studies from the University of Hawai'i at Mānoa, continued. "Performing those ceremonies of worship, like reciting a prayer before entering the forest in order to pay respect to all of the deities who helped the trees grow, is what allowed them to live so sustainably for more than a thousand years without any contact from Westerners in the most isolated landmass on Earth."

Hearing the passion in Anela's voice, I began to think about Betty, and her insistence that the cousins worship the Hawaiian sun gods at least once a day. Back then, I thought that Betty just really liked the sun, but now I knew that there was more to the story. As a lover of all parts of Hawaiian culture, Betty understood what Hawaiians believe to be true: There is a living spirit attached to all aspects of nature. She, too, believed in the spirit of the ocean, and the spirit of the wind, and the spirit of the sun. But for Hawaiians, that belief is even more profound, because it is tied directly back to their own ancestors. Aloha 'āina is a heartfelt love for the very land that made their ancestors' survival possible—and a communal sense of responsibility to care for it so that it may continue to sustain them in the present and the future.

"It is a lifestyle that is foundational to the Hawaiian way of thinking," Anela continued. "It teaches us that, as Hawaiians, we have a familial relationship to the environment. It is prevalent in the way we carry ourselves and in our actions and in our consciousness." And it's also one that Anela and many of her fellow Hawaiians try to practice every day by always being considerate of the environment, whether that's through actions as simple as conserving water by taking shorter showers, making sure lights are turned off when exiting a room, and eliminating single-use plastics, or larger actions like planting native trees

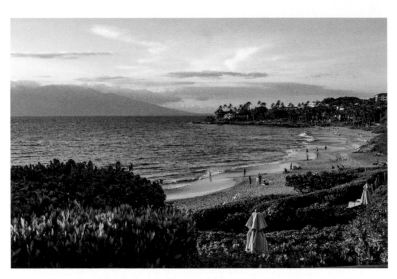

Maui: Hawaiians are mindful about caring for their environment in part so they don't ever lose views like this.

in areas that have been deforested, and leaving a place cleaner than they found it.

After we parted ways, Anela emailed me a poem from Joseph Nāwahī, a prominent Hawaiian author, historian, and scholar from the late 1800s, to help further explain the concept of aloha ʻāina. He described it as the "magnetic pull" that is tied to ancestral lands and exists in the heart of every Hawaiian, guiding his or her everyday practice:

> That is what the heart of a Hawaiian feels for his own native land. His aloha cannot be seen, held, or felt; but it is widespread, and it points inevitably to the land of his ancestors, just like the needle of a compass.

Later that evening, I sat outside on my balcony in my hotel room to re-read the poem. In many ways, I realized, Hawaiians are among the world's original sustainability experts, having developed an intuitive understanding of the environment long before scientific reasoning came along. Sure, they had traveled to the islands with select plants and animals from Polynesia—taro, 'uala (sweet potato), noni, chickens, and pigs, to name a few—and they'd brought a couple stories and chants with them, too. One of them, the honi, in which people exchange ha (the breath of life) and mana (spiritual energy) by putting their foreheads and noses together and inhaling at the same time when they meet, is still practiced to this day. But otherwise, the ancient Hawaiians had nothing but the land, their 'āina. They developed complex systems of irrigation and fishing and navigation, in addition to cultivating that spiritual relationship with nature that Anela described. All of this enabled them to live in complete harmony with the land ('āina) and the ocean (kai or moana) and each other for centuries.

AND YET, LIKE MANY INDIGENOUS CULTURES AROUND THE WORLD, NATIVE HAWAIIANS HAVE AN UNJUST AND HEARTBREAKING HISTORY OF OPPRESSION.

Once Hawai'i was colonized by the Europeans, and the Natives' land was taken away, they were forced to adapt to Western ways. And that's a big part of the reason why oral storytelling and oral tradition plays such a significant role in Hawaiian cultural history. Since the Europeans didn't believe that Hawaiian knowledge should be taught, passing it down orally was the only way for Hawaiians to preserve their native language and their ancient wisdom. "Our stories and our language and our traditions are part of us," Anela had told me earlier that afternoon. "If we lose them, we lose who we are."

E Ola Ka Ōlelo Hawai'i
(The Hawaiian Language Shall Live)

The Hawaiian language nearly reached extinction as a result of colonialism. Fortunately, during the Hawaiian Renaissance of the 1970s—a movement to revitalize the true Hawaiian identity— activists pushed to reclaim and revive the language, and it's on the upswing to this day. But the tumultuous history of the Hawaiian language still represents the larger story of Hawaiian oppression through the centuries—which continues today. Here's a brief timeline.

FIFTH CENTURY CE: Polynesian settlers sailed to the Hawaiian islands.

1778: British explorer Captain James Cook and his crew arrived in Hawai'i and recorded the Hawaiian language for the first time on the island of Kaua'i. Up until then, it was only spoken, not documented.

1795: King Kamehameha the Great established the Kingdom of Hawai'i, a monarchy in which all of the Hawaiian Islands were united under one government.

1820: American Christian missionaries arrived in Hawai'i to spread their ideas and "civilize" the Native Hawaiians.

1826: The missionaries converted the Hawaiian language from oral to written, standardizing the Hawaiian alphabet so that they could communicate the messages of the Bible to the Hawaiian people.

1855: The first of many contract workers arrived from Asia to work on Hawai'i's sugar plantations. A form of broken Hawaiian, 'ōlelo pa'i'ai, was used on the plantations.

1893: A group of missionaries and foreign residents overthrew the Kingdom of Hawai'i with a coup d'état against Queen Lili'uokalani.

1896: The Hawaiian language was entirely banned from schools and from the government—and English became the official language. Teachers were told they would be fired for speaking Hawaiian to their students, and children were told they would be punished for speaking Hawaiian as well.

1898: President William McKinley annexed Hawai'i to the United States. A new language called Pidgin, or Hawai'i Creole English, was developed when Hawaiians without access to English in their daily lives were forced to mix English words with Hawaiian pronunciation and other influences from plantation immigrants.

1919: A law was passed that required the Hawaiian language to be taught as a "foreign language," though the law was poorly enforced by the Department of Education.

1957: The Hawaiian dictionary by linguists Mary Kawena Pukui and Samuel H. Elbert was published, making Hawaiian accessible to younger generations. This dictionary is considered the key to the rebirth of the Hawaiian language to this day.

1959: Under President Dwight D. Eisenhower, Hawai'i became the fiftieth state in America, much to the dismay of many Native Hawaiians, who remained loyal to the Kingdom of Hawai'i.

1970s: The Hawaiian Renaissance emerged as an antidote to the stereotypical tiki-and-grass-skirts tourism culture that had previously reigned. With this renaissance came a renewed appreciation for the Hawaiian language.

1972: University of Hawai'i professor Larry Kimura started a radio show called *Ka Leo Hawai'i* that featured a different Native speaker each week. NPR later called this the show that sparked the Hawaiian-language revival.

1978: Hawaiian became the official language of Hawai'i once more, and the study of Hawaiian was promoted by the state.

1987: The Hawai'i Department of Education began to fund public all-Hawaiian-language-immersion schools—where courses are taught in Hawaiian until fifth grade, at which point English is gradually introduced—after a group of private Hawaiian immersion preschools began the movement. Many people view this as one of the most successful revivals of an indigenous language in modern history.

2007: The University of Hawai'i at Hilo offered a doctoral degree in Hawaiian and Indigenous Language and Culture Revitalization—the first doctorate in the world to revitalize an indigenous language.

2013: The 26th Legislature of the State of Hawai'i passed education legislation that included the phrase "in Hawai'i's two official languages" for the first time.

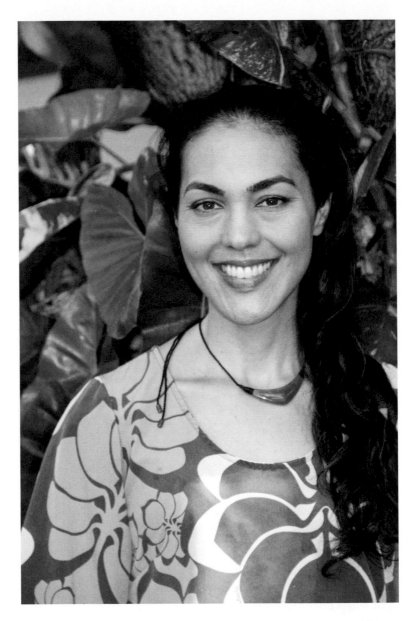

Lanai: Cultural practitioner Anela Evans surrounded by her beloved 'āina.

A few days after I chatted with Anela, I took the ferry back to Maui to talk story with another cultural preservationist, Kala Baybayan Tanaka. I'd been thinking a lot about the role that storytelling plays in our greater health and well-being since my chat with Anela, and was feeling inspired to talk to my parents and my grandparents and my aunts and uncles about my own upbringing. Before my trip, I wouldn't have thought that calling my dad to ask him about his childhood could play such a prominent role in my own well-being, but my short time in Hawai'i had already taught me otherwise. The minute I touched down in Maui and told my airport taxi driver that I was a writer looking into Hawaiian wellness, he even said, "Ah yes, so you're coming to talk to our kupunas (the Hawaiian word for elders) then!" I loved how he intuitively knew I wasn't there for the beachside fitness classes or the açai bowls or the Kava (a traditional herbal drink found on the menu at many Hawai'i health bars). Hawaiians have deep respect for their elders and their wisdom, and, like so many locals, he understood the connection between the past and the present as the key to well-being.

As the education coordinator for Hui O Wa'a Kaulua—a nonprofit dedicated to the practice and perpetuation of Hawaiian canoe building and the art and science of wayfinding—Kala is one of the leaders of a movement to revive the ancient Polynesian tradition of navigation. When the Polynesians originally sailed to the Hawaiian islands on double-hulled canoes back in the fifth century CE, they used only the stars and the wind and the ocean swells to guide them—no tools or instruments of any kind. These wayfinding techniques have been passed down through oral tradition, from a master to an apprentice, for centuries, but they were almost forgotten in Hawaiʻi during all of those years of cultural oppression. Kala is determined to never let that happen again—especially because she feels most at peace when she's out there on the waves.

"The preservation of navigation techniques is part of our identity as Hawaiians," she told me over lunch on the beach in South Maui. It was one of those postcard-perfect days that people associate with Hawaiʻi, where all I could hear was the gentle waves lapping on the shoreline coupled with the sweet melodies of traditional Hawaiian folk music playing softly in the background, and I felt so honored to be spending it with one of the island's most respected humans. ("You're going to love Kala" was a common reply when I told people I was meeting her.)

"Voyaging is what makes us unique, and it is a huge contributor in my solidity in knowing who I am," she continued. Like her ancestors before her, Kala can *feel* the tiniest shift of an ocean swell, and *hear* the direction of the wind changing ever so slightly. Those little notes, while seemingly insignificant to those not trained to listen for them, tell her everything she needs to know—and her ability to hear them is a fundamental part of her identity. "When I'm out there on the canoe, I feel like I'm not alone, because I'm surrounded by all of my ancestors. It's an assuring and spiritual feeling, a feeling of belonging, a feeling that I know who I am because I know where I come from," she told me, echoing Greg's initial "know your story" sentiment. "Even in a world that's always changing, I'm looking at the same stars they used to guide them, I'm sailing the same sea roads they sailed, and I'm experiencing all sorts of forces of nature, just as they did. To me, the canoe is that connector that brings me closer to my past and present place in space."

It was becoming clearer and clearer to me that connecting to your roots through the act of storytelling and cultural preservation is a quintessential part of Hawaiian wellness. But Kala also told me that preserving the *philosophy* of navigation is equally important—and it turns out, that philosophy is filled with wisdom, too.

ANCIENT HAWAIIANS BELIEVED IN LETTING LIFE "REVEAL ITSELF" TO YOU.

When the ancient Hawaiians first left Tahiti to sail to Hawai'i, they hadn't actually seen the Hawaiian islands before— but they knew land was there because of migratory birds that only feed on land. They observed a couple species of such birds— including the kōlea and the plover—leave and return annually in the same direction, and these comings and goings all acted as important clues that there was land. That's where the philosophy comes in: Ancient Hawaiians learned to trust early on that there was more to see than meets the eye.

"One of the most powerful things that my navigating elders told me in my learning was, 'You don't have to see the island to know that it is there,'" Kala told me. "In the beginning of my learning as a voyager, I was so fixated on being the first one to see the island. I had to see the island. Sometimes I think too much from a perspective of Western thinking, [when really] we need to shift and honor the diversity the indigenous cultural perspectives show us when it comes to how we know what's there. It's not always physical. There are clues like the birds, and the color of the clouds, and volcanic smoke, and fish, and the smell of the island. The superpower that my kupuna and all people have, if they just took the time to develop it, is the power to be super observers. We can all be super observers if we want to."

We can also use this power of observation to change the way we look at the world, I learned. "The original Hawaiian way of thinking, the Oceanic way of thinking that we're trying to preserve, is that you're not going to Tahiti—Tahiti is going to come to *you*," Kala continued. Her ancestors tuned into their surroundings to get their bearings, which is why you'll hear Hawaiians today talk about things "revealing themselves" to you.

"It's a simple, very non-Western way of thinking, one that has helped me realize that things don't have to be so complicated," Kala explained. "More will come to you and reveal itself when you are calm and clearheaded—and that applies in and out of the water. If you're worried about where you're going, your mind focuses on that fear. But if you just take the time to be still and listen, you'll be more likely to hear the wind and the stars and the ocean swells telling you where you are. We believe that you just have to listen and observe and feel the call of the mana (energy), and it will come."

Given the importance of conversation in Hawaiian culture, I wasn't surprised to learn that Hawaiians place equal emphasis on the art of listening. In fact, a couple days later, while chatting with Maui-based kumu lauhala (weaving teacher) Pi'iali'i Lawson, I learned that it's part of a greater Hawaiian philosophy known as "nānā ka maka; ho'olohe ka pepeiao; pa'a ka waha." This translates to "observe with your eyes, listen with your ears, and quiet your mouth." Most Hawaiians learn this concept at a young age, as many kumus—teachers or "sources of knowledge"—teach without words. Instead, they ask that their students simply observe and listen and then follow suit—an idea that continues to impact the way that they view and operate in the world moving forward. "What we're really doing by keeping this concept in mind is learning to fully immerse ourselves into whatever we are doing, and to trust ourselves as well as the process, both physical and spiritual," Pi'iali'i told me. "When we ask questions in the middle of the teaching, we are interrupting our learning process, and it's often because of our impatience and lack of trust in ourselves. Following this practice in and outside of weaving challenges us to listen to what is going on so we can learn—because all we need to know is being presented and revealed right in front of us."

As Kala said, this idea of things "revealing themselves" to us is a *very* non-Western way of approaching the world. Think about it: In our rise-and-grind culture, we're encouraged to go for what we want. Word on the street is that we can hustle our way to our dreams, that with a little self-optimization—all things that enable us to work harder, better, faster, and stronger—we can conquer the world. While this isn't always true, thanks to racism and classism that unfairly limits many from the start, a large majority of Westerners are encouraged to push, strive, and thrive until we have made our dreams happen. Rather than tuning into our surroundings for guidance, we remain convinced that we need to plow on forward until we actually *see* the land, because we control our own destinies. What Kala and Pi'iali'i's ancient Hawaiian ancestors seemed to be asking was: Do we, though? What if we trusted that, by listening to the signs all around us, we would still get where we need to go? What if we chilled for a minute and let things reveal themselves to us? Americans are not very good at not knowing—but what if we stopped trying to plan it all out?

On my final day in Maui, I took a long late-afternoon stroll on the beach to mull over what I'd learned. This philosophy of nānā ka maka; hoʻolohe ka pepeiao; paʻa ka waha had really resonated with me. Isn't it nice to think that if you do everything you can to get yourself into the metaphorical canoe, and you silence your inner worries and just *listen*, and *observe*, that the wind and the water may just take care of the rest? As I waded through the surf, flip-flops in hand, I started thinking about how the navigational philosophy applied to my own life. Rahul and I had been together for more than five years at that point, and we had a lot of choices to make in the near future about family, work, and where to live. I'd been getting sucked into the "what is our life plan" vacuum lately, and as I looked out over the ocean, the waves sparkling in the golden-hour light, I made a pact with myself: I'd try to let life reveal itself to me even more in the coming years. I did not have to have everything figured out. Standing there feeling the warm salt water of the Pacific wash over my toes, the same salt water that ancient Hawaiians had sailed through thousands of years ago, and the same salt water that ran through Betty's veins, I reminded myself to take a deep breath and just chill. All I had to do was get myself into the canoe and listen—and soon enough I'd know the way.

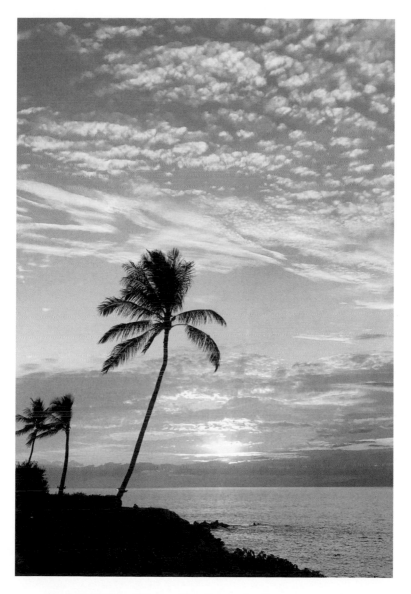

Maui: If only life could reveal itself to me in this setting every day.

Soothe Your Spirit with Hi'uwai, the Hawaiian Saltwater Cleanse

Because of their spiritual relationship with water, many Hawaiians perform a hi'uwai—a cleansing ritual that takes place in the ocean or a stream—when they feel stressed. There are thousands of different types of hi'uwais, all of which serve a different purpose and have been passed down through oral tradition in Hawaiian families for centuries. "Hi'uwais are directly connected to our health and well-being, as the process allows us to move forward with our days and lives from the many physical and spiritual forces that may be holding us down or back," Pi'iali'i told me.

Most families have different hi'uwais. "Because our ancestors have been practicing these basic healing methods for generations, doing one is really comforting," added Lokahi Oriana, an O'ahu-based jewelry maker. Here are a few for you to try:

To release something from the past:

Walk into the ocean with leaves from a plant that's special to you. Hawaiians use the ki plant, also referred to as the ti plant, which early Hawaiians believed had great spiritual power. (It's one of the ancient "canoe plants"—plants originally brought to Hawai'i by the ancient Polynesians.) Then say a prayer, tear up each leaf piece by piece, and scatter the pieces in the water, with each piece meant to represent something you want to release.

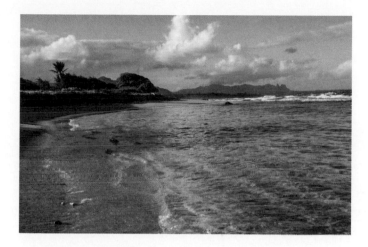

For good luck:

Take something important to you into the ocean early in the morning to wash away any bad spirits. Many Hawaiian tattoo artists who practice kakau—the ancient Polynesian method of hand-tapping, in which designs are hand-tapped onto the skin—bring their tools into the ocean each morning to bless them.

If you don't live near the ocean:

No problem—many Hawaiians even carry a small bag of paʻakai (Hawaiian sea salt) with them in their pockets at all times, in case they feel the need to purify their spirits or clear their heads but aren't by the sea. Just take a pinch of salt, put it under your tongue, and let it dissolve. "Sea salt is cleansing for many cultures, and it's a great tool to carry with you," Piʻialiʻi told me. "It serves the same purpose and symbolizes cleansing and purification when done with the right intention."

As I was planning my trip to Hawaiʻi, the Big Island started making headlines across the globe. Since 2009, a group called the Thirty Meter Telescope International Observatory has been planning to build a $1.5 billion Thirty Meter Telescope (TMT) on top of Maunakea, a dormant volcano on the island that's home to the highest peak in the entire state of Hawaiʻi. Astronomers believe that Maunakea's location makes it one of the best spots to study the sky and the origins of the universe in the entire world, and they have already built thirteen smaller telescopes on its peak. But if the TMT gets built, scientists say it will provide an even better opportunity to observe the formation of new stars, planets, and galaxies than the telescopes that are already there—not to mention bring lots of money and jobs to the island.

The majority of Native Hawaiians are not on board with this plan. Why would they be? While most say they are not anti-science, they *are* against building the TMT on "the Mauna," as they call it, because they consider it to be one of the most sacred spots in the entire archipelago chain. When the Polynesian settlers first sailed to the islands, they named Maunakea for the god of creation Wakea—the Sky Father—since it's the closest physical piece of land to Him in the sky. Hawaiians believe that this is a place where humans can enter heaven, which is why they feel that building telescopes there is especially sacrilegious. Throughout history, the mountain was used as a burial ground for their most sacred ancestors.

Just a few weeks before I was to arrive on the islands, the growing tension between the Native Hawaiians and the Thirty Meter Telescope International Observatory reached an all-time high when a group of twenty-eight Hawaiian kupunas (wise, respected elders) were arrested on the weekend that construction of the TMT was supposed to officially begin. In a powerful protest statement, they'd joined together to form a line blocking the access road to Maunakea, which is the only road construction workers can take to get up to the telescopes. This news made waves on a global scale, as it was one of the first times in history that a group of elders united and took to the front lines in such a prominent way.

The kupunas quickly became heroes—and the Maunakea story came to represent so much more than the telescope as a result. It became a symbol of the marginalization the majority of indigenous cultures around the world have faced and continue to face in the wake of colonization, and of the fight to revive their cultures. Although Hawai'i is often named the happiest state in the nation on all sorts of lists (most recently, by the personal-finance website WalletHub in September 2019), many Native Hawaiians—who make up only 20 percent of the population in Hawai'i overall—struggle with mental health issues. Like in many indigenous cultures around the world, domestic violence, depression, and suicide have developed as a result of feeling forgotten and disconnected from who they really are. Today, there are only about one thousand Native Hawaiian speakers left, the majority of whom live on Ni'ihau, the privately owned island that's the last community of full-blooded Hawaiians. (An additional eight thousand Hawaiians can speak and understand their native language fluently.) One old Hawaiian textbook called *Nānā i Ke Kumu*, published in 1972—thirteen years after Hawaiʻi became an official state in the US—explains this loss of identity:

> *The Hawaiian lived for many years isolated from the rest of the world, with a viable culture that met the needs of a thriving, industrious and religious people. Then came the foreigner with his technology and Judeo-Christian culture. He saw the native beliefs as pagan and inferior, and superimposed his culture. In order to gain acceptance, avoid ridicule and disapproval, the Hawaiian gradually adapted to Western ways. However, he secretly hung on to some of the beliefs and ways of his own culture. The confusion in his sense of identity which resulted exists today.*

After reading news story after news story about Maunakea, I realized that my trip was coming along at an incredibly historic time in Hawaiian history. So I changed my itinerary around and added in a last-minute trip to Maunakea in order to better understand the preservation battle in the making—and the spirit of aloha that seemed to be pulsing through the islands. Thanks to the kupunas' epic, visible stand to reclaim their land and their culture, Maunakea had become an international symbol of hope.

———

I hadn't been back to the Big Island since I was fifteen, and I had all sorts of thoughts running through my head when I landed: Would it still look the same? Would I feel like a teenager again? Would the air still smell a little bit like plumeria mixed with volcanic ash? And perhaps most importantly: What would the energy feel like with all of the Maunakea happenings? My answers were yes, no, yes, and . . . buzzing.

Many locals and travelers alike believe that the Big Island—which is largely barren and dotted with black-sand volcanic rock beaches from a famous volcanic eruption in 1801—may just be the most spiritual of all the islands, thanks in large part to the presence of sacred Maunakea. Spend some time in a cafe or bar in Kona or Hilo, the Big Island's two biggest cities, and you'll no doubt hear people talking about how the island "called" to them more than the others, or how they felt its magnetic pull. I took a yoga class in Maui, and my teacher told me that he can hardly even go to the Big Island because he feels such intense pangs of emotion while he's there.

Granted, I associate the island with my family, so I am a bit biased in my love for its spirit, but I agree—there's definitely a *there* there. An energy. You can feel it in the soft air that wraps around you like a blanket, and in the moon and the stars that shine so brightly; it's possible to walk on the beach in the middle of the night and still see. On my first night in Kona, I gazed up at the sky and thought of my favorite *Calvin and Hobbes* comic strip, where six-year-old Calvin looks up at the starry night and shouts, "I'm significant!" And then, in the next panel: ". . . screamed the dust speck." The Big Island is the kind of place that makes you think about how much of a dust speck you really are.

I was nervous to head up to Maunakea from Kona on my second day. I was, after all, heading to a place of protest: Would I be safe? And would I be welcome as an outsider? I calmed myself down by taking comfort in the excitement many locals around all of the various islands had shown about my journey. Lots of them had been raving about Kapu Aloha, which is the non-violent code of conduct that had been issued by the kupunas. The code of conduct means that you aren't allowed to swear, drink alcohol, or use drugs or violence of any kind on the Mauna—and most importantly, you must stay positive. If you feel yourself getting negative, it's your kuleana (responsibility) to leave the Mauna.

"Kapu Aloha is all about peace, love, and happiness," Iko Balanga, a much-loved waterman on the Big Island, had told me on the beach the day before. (*Waterman* is the local term for someone who understands the ways of the ocean through knowledge often passed down from generation to generation.) Iko has felt one with the waves his entire life and now runs his own ocean adventure company called Anelakai Adventures.

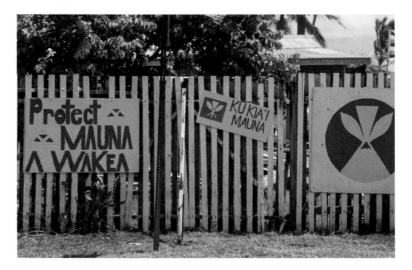

Kauaʻi: Maunakea signs appeared on all the islands, not just the Big Island.

"When you're up there on the Mauna, you'll see how positive it is—it'll make you live forever. If you live with Kapu Aloha, you'll be happy and healthy for the rest of your life."

When I arrived, it was cold and windy. Not cold by East Coast standards, but cold by Hawai'i standards: I had to put on long pants, a down vest, and a wool hat. In Hawai'i! There were people camped out on the side of the road, carrying signs that said things like, "Aloha Will Save the World," and "Road Closed Due to Desecration," and "Aloha 'aina." My favorite one was, "We Are Protectors, Not Protestors." As soon as I saw that sign, I quickly lectured myself for thinking I was coming to a place of protest in the first place. The gathering was as far from a protest as could be—it was a spiritual movement.

The kia'i (protectors) who'd come to the Mauna from all of the Hawaiian islands had already been camped up there for seventy-one days when I got there. And boy, had they set up shop. There was a food tent, a kupuna tent especially reserved for the wise elders, and even a programming schedule that highlighted the four special ceremonies per day—one small sunrise ceremony, followed by three larger ones at 8 a.m., noon, and 5:30 p.m.—all done free of charge out of the goodness of aloha. Multiple Hawaiian-studies professors and doctors had even quit their jobs so they could help run the movement and take care of the kupuna each day. During the ceremonies—referred to as *protocols*—the protectors all gathered together in the middle of the Maunakea Access Road to chant and speak and dance the hula, which is another way in which Hawaiians honor their culture and connect to their ancestors.

I joined for the noon protocol. We did some call-and-response chanting, a couple people stood up and gave blessings and offerings to Maunakea (one woman gave a coconut followed by a chant), and then we all joined together to do the hula right there in the middle of the road. Though I felt a little nervous to dance at first, the leaders were so encouraging and so grateful that we were all there that my inhibitions evaporated quickly. And I was also inspired by an Oʻahu man named Michael, who'd given a speech thanking Hawaiians for their knowledge before we started dancing. Though not a Hawaiian himself, he's lived on the islands for years and had been driving Hawaiians to the airport in Oʻahu for free for the past seventy-one days if they told him they were flying to the Big Island for the Mauna. "I'm terrified of public speaking," he began, "but I was drawn to come up here to let you all know how much I love you and support you. All of the real knowledge I have ever gained in life I have learned from the Hawaiians." He started crying during his speech, tears of appreciation and gratitude, and I nearly did, too.

Hawaiians have been oppressed for generations, forced to give up their own culture and leave their own land in the hands of developers. The cost of living has risen so high that many Native Hawaiians have moved to Las Vegas—now dubbed "the ninth island"—where it's more affordable and they can still get jobs in the hospitality industry, the trade many locals are trained in. And yet, despite all of this hardship, they are still out there fighting the good fight with smiles on their faces and aloha in their hearts. The Kapu Aloha was overpowering.

As it was getting colder and colder and my day on the Mauna was winding down, I spotted one of the most active and

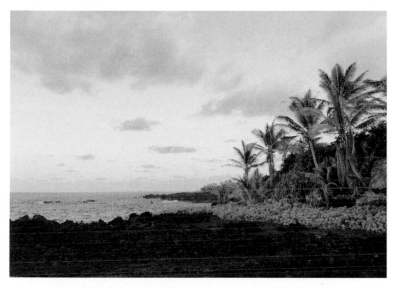

Hana, Maui: Hawaiians believe that everything you see here
is connected—and that's aloha.

well-known kupunas, who was a head professor of Hawaiian
knowledge at one of the public universities. I'd been working up
the courage to ask him for an interview all day, but he'd been
so busy running the show that I hadn't gotten the chance until
now.

"Excuse me?" I said as I tapped him on the shoulder. "I'm
Annie, a journalist from New York, and I was wondering if you
have a couple minutes to chat with me about how Maunakea is
changing the face of Hawai'i," I said. I thought it was a solid
intro: short and to the point. But the professor had another
direction in mind.

"You shouldn't be trying to interview anyone," he replied
gently. "The story, instead, is this." He paused to gesture to the
surrounding crowd. "The story is that this is happening. Look

around! The story is that this place exists," he told me with a proud smile. "People are out here, working so hard to make all of this programming happen, camping out in the cold—and no one is getting paid. This is all done because of Kapu Aloha. Kapu Aloha is your story."

As a journalist, I figured he'd want to get the word out, so I was fairly surprised that he didn't want to chat for longer. But after I thanked him for his time, I realized he was right. The entire setup at Maunakea *was* the word. Locals had flown in from all of the islands, quit their jobs, given up their paychecks, and camped outside in the cold for seventy-one days to protect their precious land—all while channeling positivity through their non-violent actions. Iko, the waterman I'd interviewed, had told me that he'd never seen anything like it before in history. He called it the start of a second Hawaiian Renaissance, and I understood then just how right he was. Standing there on the Mauna, soaking it all in one more time before getting in my car to head home, I thought about all of the Hawaiians I'd met on my travels, who'd taught me so much about their ancestral wisdom. I thought of the navigators, the weavers, the cultural practitioners, and now, the protectors . . . all of the Hawaiians working together to build a better future by preserving their past.

On the mainland, it's hard to find "good vibes only" culture in its pure form. Even the people who are spreading the good word are often entwined in the hustle culture, selling a "just breathe" tank top to go with the wisdom. But in Hawai'i, this message is more deeply ingrained, thanks to the ancestral lessons that Hawaiians have worked tirelessly to preserve over thousands of years. "Girl, we've been on these tips for *generations*!" Uilani Bobbit, the Hawaiian-language professor who explained the deeper meaning of aloha earlier, had told me over coffee one afternoon in O'ahu. We were talking about all things wellness and how something as simple as walking barefoot could become a trend with its own title: *grounding*.

"We've always walked barefoot on the Earth because we've always understood the importance of connecting with the 'āina. This is nothing new to us. But people in the twenty-first century are just 'finding out' about these concepts now!" she'd exclaimed. What everyone can learn from the ancient Hawaiian wisdom, she'd continued, is that nothing is ever going to change unless you change your spiritual form. "And the best way to do that is to go back to the source, back to your roots, whatever they may be. Back to the original idea of aloha. I really think that aloha is the only thing that will heal the world. It's inside all of us, in our spirits and our souls. We just have to access what's already there."

"Even if we're not Hawaiian?" I'd asked her.

"Yes, aloha is in all of us, Hawaiian or not," she'd replied. "Remember, it's really about connection. Saying aloha means that you understand there's a connection between everything. Our ancestors knew that, which is how they were able to survive for so long in isolation. I am not any more important than the tree because I *am* the tree. I am this dirt, I am this butterfly, I am this plant. Problems happen when we don't recognize that we are all the same thing in different forms. So can we just work on recognizing that we're all connected? That's what the world needs."

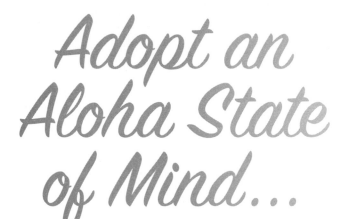

Adopt an Aloha State of Mind...

WHEREVER YOU ARE

Soak in the knowledge of your elders.

Ask your parents or your grandparents or your older neighbors about their lives before you were born: What are some traditions or tips they think should be passed down to future generations? It's not about understanding your technical ancestral lineage through genetic testing—it's about knowing your story by making the time to connect to the elders who helped shape your path. The process of listening to and passing along stories gives meaning to our lives.

Take care of the land around you.

Aloha 'āina (the love of the land) is a central philosophy of Hawaiian thought. To weave it into your daily life, do everything you can to take care of the environment that sustains you. Professor Bobbit also suggests "humbling yourself and asking permission in your vibes" before you enter a natural space that's not your own.

Be patient.

Is there a part of your life that you're forcing into being? Rather than pushing to make it happen, try letting life reveal itself to you instead. You may end up with something better and more suited to your soul than what you dreamed up for yourself in the first place.

Tap into the power of rituals.

Traditions (like performing hiʻuwais and making and giving lei on special occasions) help Hawaiians feel closer to their history and to themselves. Is there a similarly meaningful ritual you can do that connects you to your roots or shows your loved ones you care?

Remember that we are all connected.

This is the true essence of the aloha spirit. We are all sharing the same breath, the breath of life. And the more we recognize that connection, the closer we'll be to worldwide well-being.

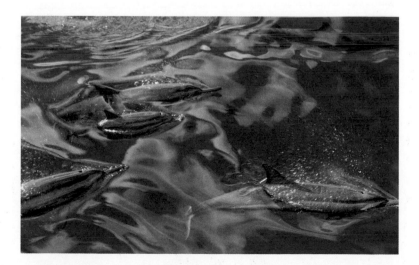

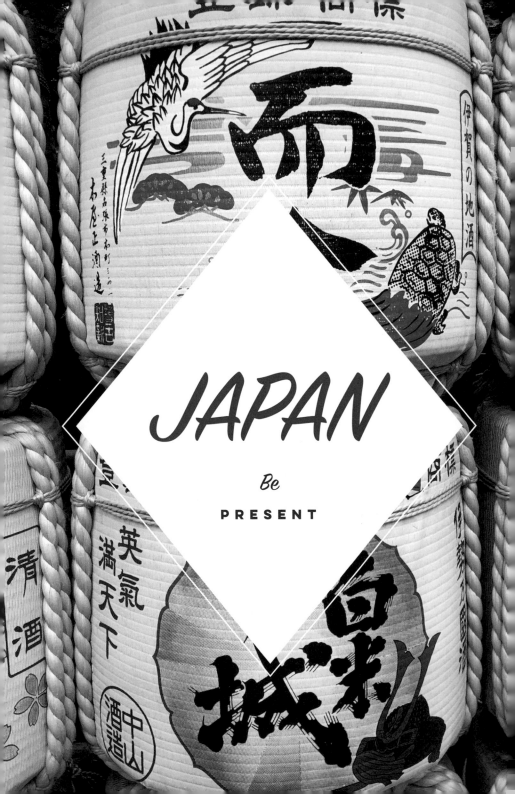

JAPAN

Be

PRESENT

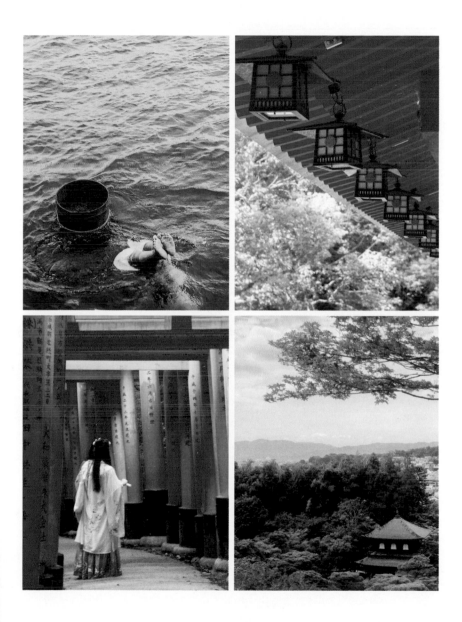

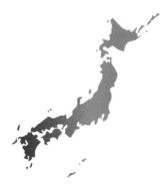

*T*HE FIRST THING I noticed about hiking in Japan is that there weren't that many Japanese people hiking in Japan.

I was there on a two-week group trekking trip from Kyoto to Tokyo that took us along various routes including the Kumano Kodo, a series of ancient pilgrimage trails through the Kii Mountain Range in rural Japan. I'm generally not a fan of the idea of a "bucket-list" trip (traveling itself is epic no matter where you go!), but those who are often put this hike on the top of the list. Once a sacred trail reserved for Buddhist monks and other religious pilgrims on a quest to reach some of Japan's most sacred shrines and temples, the Kumano Kodo was originally designed to be a religious journey all its own. The terrain is rocky and mountainous, and the idea back then was that simply making it through was a way to experience the area's sacred spirit. Today, it's open to all explorers who, like me, want to challenge themselves with a difficult hike and visit three of Japan's most sacred shrines (together known as Kumano Sanzan).

When I'd gotten the invitation to go on the trip months earlier, I'd been ecstatic. Like many people just trying to get by in today's hyper-prompt world, I'd been feeling overwhelmed by all of the usual suspects—busyness, disconnection, all of the on-ness—and I was struggling to operate with grace without abruptly exploding. My life had devolved into a never-ending deluge of emails and text messages that required a near-instant response, and I'd somehow found myself starting emails with "Sorry for my delay!" if I hadn't responded within two hours. I was drained by feeling both constantly behind and constantly worried about the future at the same time—and the peacefulness of rural Japan seemed like a great place to get myself back to the present. To learn about how to truly be present.

I heard about the *idea* of being present all the time in New York. I heard about it from my breathy, love-and-light yoga teachers, who insisted we all take a deep inhale to connect with our core essence, and from my Instagram feed, which had somehow become a digital hub of new-age spirituality, and even from some of the brands I worked with at the wellness magazine, who wanted consumers to associate their products with the concept of the here and now. But that was the whole thing: I'd heard about it too much. *Presence* and *patience* had become words people just threw around—but none of it had actually resonated. Right away, rural Japan, with its quiet forests and its bamboo stillness, seemed like a more authentic and genuine antidote to all of the go-go-go noise.

My hiking guide, Keigo, a soft-spoken fifty-something man with kind eyes and a gentle disposition, told me that there weren't many Japanese people on the Kumano Kodo because locals in Japan tend to stick to shorter hikes, not days-long treks. "We Japanese are actually a bit lazy in terms of physical activities," he laughed. "Nowadays, you can just take a bus to the Three Grand Shrines of Kumano, so most Japanese people just do that to get the spiritual experience." From there, Keigo and I started chatting about all sorts of other differences between my expectations of Japan and the actual reality of it. And once he knew that I was interested in chatting about such topics, he shared all sorts of additional thoughts and local knowledge with me throughout the trip.

WELLNESS IN JAPAN, I LEARNED, IS A COMPLICATED SUBJECT.

It's no secret that Westerners tend to associate Japan with spiritual enlightenment. Despite the fact that this is certainly a romanticized idea of Japan, the country is still a well-being mecca for the searchers and the seekers of the world. People love to read and talk about Japanese lifestyle concepts like ikigai, the idea that finding your sense of purpose or reason for living leads to true happiness, and kintsugi, the idea that we can turn our scars into beauty, based on the Japanese practice of repairing broken pottery with gold. Organizing expert Marie Kondo, who taught the world how to tidy up and get rid of things that don't spark joy, is super popular here in the West. And who can forget about the incredibly healthy seniors in Okinawa? Japan has the longest life expectancy rate in the entire world, and Okinawa—a group of about twenty-four islands—has the largest concentration of those centenarians (people who live to a hundred years old or more). As one of journalist Dan Buettner's five Blue Zones—places around the globe where people live the longest—Okinawa has become a hot spot for Westerners looking to Japan for longevity secrets.

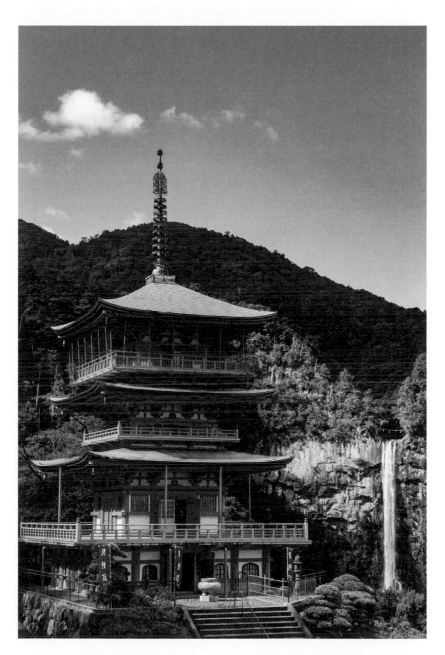
Kumano Nachi Taishai: The last grand shrine of the Kumano Kodo.

Because the country is known for its ancient wellness wisdom, it's easy to assume that its residents are still tapping into those lessons in their daily lives. But while some of those philosophies have stood the test of time—like wabi-sabi, the art of finding beauty in imperfection—many other Japanese wellness concepts have not. The modern world has hit Japan hard. For all of its deeply rooted wellness history, Japan paradoxically has a very high rate of stress today. In fact, working hours throughout the country were once so long that, in April 2019, the Japanese government instituted a work-style reform bill that limited employee overtime to 80 hours per month. This came after previous surveys found that nearly one quarter of Japanese companies require their employees to work more than that.

Death by overwork, known as *karoshi*—in which employees either take their own lives or suffer from a stress-related heart attack or stroke—is fortunately on the decline, but it does still exist. While the deep-seated gaman philosophy, defined as "enduring the seemingly unbearable with patience and dignity," was once revered in Japanese society as a model for the virtue of grit, thought leaders are now saying that it's part of the reason why some Japanese are working themselves to death. Taught to grin and bear it, to just put their heads down and keep plowing away, many Japanese are now cracking, unable to handle the myriad emotional pressures that inevitably bubble up by living that way. And so, if anything, modern Japanese citizens today are often as much in need of their own ancient cultural wisdom as everyone else. "Americans tend to think of Japan as a place where everyone is so healthy all the time, and I always see all

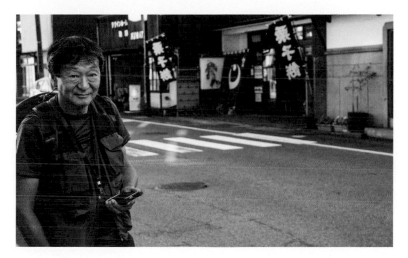

Toba: The lovely Keigo, guiding me through his country's quiet streets.

of these articles about wellness in Japanese culture," Keigo told me. "These philosophies do exist here, but really, we don't think of them in that way," he told me.

I first met my adventure group, ten other hikers from various countries in Europe, outside of our hotel in Kyoto. I'd flown to Osaka straight from Hawai'i the night before, and my first thought about Japan was the contrast between the two airports. Even though the Honolulu airport was mostly open-air, it was still loud, filled with large groups of chatty, sunburned tourists filling up on one last round of tropical cocktails. The airport in Osaka, on the other hand, was pin-drop quiet and orderly, with suitcases stacked side-by-side in neat little rows on the conveyor belt at baggage claim. Somehow even the travelers had gotten the memo to take it down a notch.

My group and I were staying at a hotel right in Kyoto's city center, and the quiet continued even there at the urban hotel. People were everywhere, yet I could still hear the birds chirping on my walk to get coffee before our meeting. *Welcome to Japan*, I thought to myself. *It really is as quiet as they say.*

After spending the first few days of our trip in Kyoto, my group and I took the train south to start our trek. In 2004, the Kumano Kodo was designated a UNESCO World Heritage Site, joining Spain's Camino de Santiago as the only other UNESCO pilgrimage trek in the entire world. There on the hike, everything modern was out of sight, out of mind, and for the next week or so, it was just us and the trees. The Japanese red cedars—also known as Japanese redwoods—towered over us, tall and majestic, some reaching up to 150 feet. There were pine trees, too, and cypress trees, and maple trees. Walking under them, I could sense that there was a clear blue sky *just* beyond the green canopy right above me, though I couldn't see it myself. Puddles of sunlight occasionally made their way through the thick umbrella of branches above me, and I would momentarily be reminded that other color palettes existed in the world. But mostly, the sky was beyond our visual reach. All I could actually see was green, and it was everywhere.

My group tended to split up during the long stretches of hiking, but I didn't feel alone at all: The forest was my hiking companion and it was teeming with life. Walking through the fresh moss-covered trees, the environment felt buzzy and moist, even though it wasn't raining, and I could hear all sorts of things moving as I walked. There were deer hopping about, and lots of birds singing. Occasionally we'd pass a stream, crystal clear and flecked with tiny sparkles, its steady trickle a welcome addition to the soundtrack. Surrounded by all of this omnipresent noise from the natural world, I felt incredibly mindful and dialed into my senses. How could I not? At one point, a huge speckled snake popped out of the cedar chips just inches in front of me, and I stopped so suddenly I nearly fell over. This was not the time to tune out. The moment was now.

BUT IT WAS ACTUALLY THE RYOKANS—NOT THE FORESTS—THAT ENDED UP TEACHING ME THE MOST ABOUT HOW TO BE PRESENT.

Most ryokans—originally called *fuseya* (free guesthouses, or a house of giving)—are in the countryside and are run by locals only. The first ryokan we stayed in sat on a small hill dotted with Tibetan prayer flags in the mountain town of Tanabe. As soon as I wobbled off the bus with my trekking backpack and heavy suitcase, I was hit with a blast of steam from the nearby onsen, which translates directly to "hot springs," but also refers to the spas built around them. Because Japan is a volcanic zone, there are more than thirty thousand onsens—all of which contain a wealth of healing minerals like sulfur, calcium, magnesium, and iron—scattered throughout its various islands. Most onsens are found in serene, natural settings, often high up in the mountains or sprinkled along the sea, which adds to their soothing appeal. On the bus ride up the mountain to Tanabe, I'd been preparing myself for the onsen's rotten-egg sulfur smell, thinking it would be overpowering, but to my surprise, it was actually lovely. The mountain air was so crisp, it seemed to wrap around the egg smell like a blanket, muting the strong sulfuric scent with its woody freshness.

The History of Ryokans

While ryokans (originally called fuseya*) have been around for centuries, they've gotten increasingly popular in recent years, especially as international travelers have become more interested in experiencing local cultures firsthand. Here's how ryokans came to be— and why they're still so steeped in tradition.*

NARA PERIOD (710-784): Ryokans were some of the first hotels in the world. They began as temporary lodging facilities within Buddhist temples as a way to help traders traveling from Edo (now Tokyo) to Kyoto's Imperial Palace actually survive their journeys. Travel was dangerous back then, with hardly any infrastructure, and many travelers were dying of starvation along Japan's highways as a result. Ryokans reflected one of the Buddhist teachings: Assisting others helps you lessen your karmic weight and accumulate merits (i.e., giving to others is good karma).

EDO PERIOD (1600s-1868): As better highways were developed, merchants began to travel more frequently, and hatagos (inns or taverns) were established along the highways as the new fuseya. But unlike the original guesthouses, they served food and charged a fee. Hatagos catered to travelers who wanted to go on a pilgrimage or visit the onsens.

MEIJI PERIOD (1868-1912): The hatagos began to decline as travelers started to take the train instead of trekking on foot. As a result, many ryokans as we know them today started to pop up near railway stations. They took their inspiration from hatagos and also from honjins, which were fancier accommodations for feudal lords.

PRESENT DAY: An onslaught of modern, luxury, amenity-heavy ryokans has been built in recent years. Even though some of them are quite over-the-top, with Michelin-starred restaurants and fancy gyms, the majority of ryokans have still managed to retain age-old customs. This includes serving kaiseki dinners (traditional multicourse meals), furnishing the guest rooms with futons, low tables, shoji (sliding paper screen doors between the sitting and sleeping areas), and tatami mats, and providing the guests with yukata (traditional cotton robes) and slippers to wear inside.

The inside of the ryokan smelled like the surrounding cedar forest, too, thanks to the customary tatami mats laid down on the floors throughout the house. Traditionally made from rice straw and the occasional wood chip, tatami mats emit a natural, earthy aroma—a pleasing reminder that you are surrounded by some of the most beautiful, unspoiled nature in the world.

Wearing regular shoes on tatami mats is considered disrespectful in Japanese culture, but two nights into my ryokan stay, I accidentally broke this crucial rule. I came back from our hike and in my rush to make it to the bathroom on time, I forgot to take off my hiking boots at the door and stepped on one of the tatami mats. Disaster! As soon as I did, two staffers rushed over to me in a panic and started pointing to my shoes, at which point I realized what I'd done. I felt beyond terrible, vowing to be more careful in the future. And I was. Things improved as I adjusted to the customs. In keeping with Japanese tradition, most ryokan guest rooms have very little furniture, just a low-to-the-ground table with two chairs without legs (basically a back rest on the floor), a tea set on the table, and a thin futon mattress with a down comforter rolled up in the corner. The staff also leaves guests a yukata—the casual, cotton version of a kimono—to wear around the ryokan and to its accompanying onsen. As the days went by, I developed a routine: come home from a long day of hiking, take my shoes off at the door, go up to my room, change into my yukata (wrapping the left side over the right, as is customary), and then . . . soak.

There is a particular magic about a post-hike onsen soak that cannot be emphasized enough. Japanese women and men have been bathing in communal onsens for centuries, using them to socialize and also to soothe sore muscles and help tame various inflammations (sulfur is one of nature's most popular anti-inflammatory minerals). Traditionally, men and women soaked together, but now this is quite rare; most onsens have separate male and female baths. And while the majority of photos of onsens depict them as steaming outdoor baths nestled into the mountains, they actually vary in size and nature, with many of them located indoors. Some are made of wood, while others are made of stone; some are big like a swimming pool and others are small like a jacuzzi. But no matter what, they are all rich with minerals and hot enough that you can see the steam rising from the water, as if from a pond on a dewy morning. Many onsens even have floating pieces of sulfur that look like scrambled egg whites, a sign that the hot spring is extra sulfuric—and thereby extra therapeutic—that day.

Also: All bathers must soak naked. And you're required to wash yourself before soaking, too. Most onsens provide soap, shampoo, and conditioner, so you just sit on a small stool and use a handheld showerhead to do all of your lathering and rinsing before stepping into the tub. I've gotta say, I was a bit nervous about the nudity at first, but I was quickly inspired by the Japanese women who didn't even flinch when I eased my way into the steaming-hot waters. It only took me a few soaks to get on their level, swapping my initial self-consciousness for a deep sigh of relief. Eventually, all I felt upon entering were the soothing minerals seeping into my skin, melting away the knots that had formed on the rocky, woodsy trails. I became so addicted to soaking that I started setting my alarm for an hour or two before we were meant to leave the ryokan so that I could soak in the

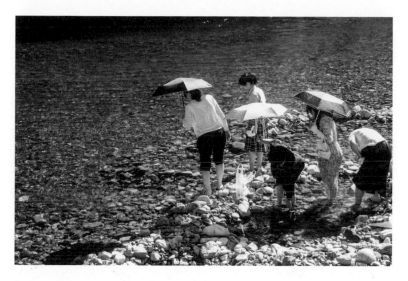

Tanabe-Shi: A group of women soak their feet in the hot springs.

morning before breakfast as well. Those morning baths tended to be a little less crowded, as onsens are traditionally taken in the evening before dinner, but I felt energized for the rest of the day after starting with a soak.

One morning, I had an especially strong revelatory moment, the kind that travelers crave, the kind that feeds and fuels our wanderlust and keeps us perpetually coming back for more. Nothing *happened*, really: I just stepped into the steaming-hot bath, one foot after the other, and stood there for a minute or two watching a pool of golden light from the sunrise pour in through the windows and catch the steam rising from the water. There was one Japanese woman at the other end of the onsen, but she barely looked up when I made that first splash with my foot. The moment was more about what *didn't* happen: My wandering mind did not wander. While I will never really

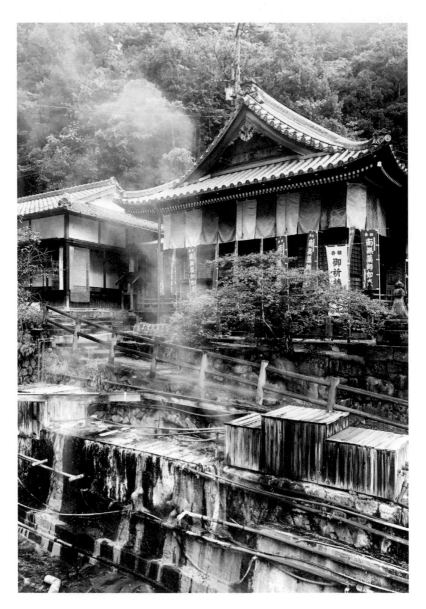

Tanabe: The steam from the onsen was impossible to miss.

know exactly how or why my fellow bather was able to stay in her own zone as I lowered myself into the hot water, pushing aside floating pieces of egg white–esque sulfur, her ability to do so inspired me. Following her lead, I took a deep breath and just . . . soaked. Later, I thought about how the Japanese, like other cultures with strong bathing traditions, have been practicing self-care since before self-care was even called self-care. Making time to soak in sulfuric water is a deeply entrenched ritual; the oldest hot spring in Japan, Dogo Onsen, dates back more than three thousand years. But in that moment, it was just me and the sulfuric steam and my content mind.

AFTER TRADITIONAL EVENING ONSEN SOAKS, IT'S USUALLY TIME FOR THE MAIN EVENT: THE POST-ONSEN FEAST. And this is where omotenashi—the term for Japanese hospitality—really shines.

Before my trip, I'd envisioned piles upon piles of sushi and ramen dinners all throughout my travels, after which I would return from Japan as one great big giant raw fish. But I quickly learned that those aren't the go-to eats in the countryside. Ryokans are centered around kaiseki, traditional multicourse dinners, followed by homemade breakfast spreads the next morning—all eaten around a low table while sitting on pillows on the floor. The kaiseki tradition honors local, seasonal ingredients that represent the surrounding area; the chefs prepare about seven or eight main dishes of regional delicacies and bring them out in ritualized stages directly after they make them, so as to maintain optimal freshness. But to call the kaiseki meals I ate *meals* is to do them a disservice. These were *feasts*. Works of art. And every one of them was extravagant. The dinners usually featured some sort of seafood—think steamed awabi (abalone), sea urchins, sashimi (sliced raw fish)—plus piping-hot noodle dishes, tempura (deep-fried vegetables, seafood, or meat), chawanmushi (soft egg custard), grilled wagyu beef, seafood hot pots, and sake. For breakfast every morning, there was some combination of white rice, miso soup, salted fish, tamagoyaki (Japanese rolled omelet), pickles, seaweed, tofu, noodles, fruit plates, green tea, and more. And although I'm embarrassed to admit that I often couldn't handle the strong smell of fish so early in the morning—waking up to the scent of seafood wafting into my room at 7 a.m. was a little too much for me, especially after multiple rounds of sake the night before—I was always in complete awe of the display of hospitality. The ryokan staff went out of their way to fix our meals and to make us feel at home.

Omotenashi enjoyed a wave of international cultural rec-ognition in 2013 when television announcer Christel Takigawa said in a speech that, if Japan was chosen as the location for the 2020 Summer Olympic Games, the Japanese would welcome the world with their hospitable spirit. Although the Tokyo Summer Olympics were postponed due to COVID-19, omotenashi is still having a moment. The philosophy has been woven into Japan's cultural fabric for centuries. While it's one of those elusive con-cepts that is hard to define, much like friluftsliv and aloha, the basic idea is that one should provide a service without expecting anything in return. It's less of a transactional service and more of a state of mind. There is no tipping in Japan because expectations for good service do not exist. It's just something that you do. It's the way you think, the way you operate in the world. Omotenashi

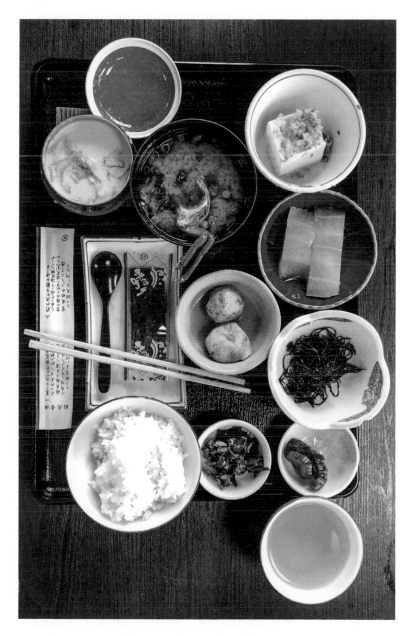

Nakatsugawa: A ryokan breakfast spread.

is about caring for others just as you care for yourself, without expecting bonus points or metaphorical "extra credit."

Exhibit A: One morning at a ryokan in the Ijika district of Toba, I realized that I needed to do laundry quite badly, so I used Google Translate to ask one of the staff members, Reiko, where the nearest laundromat was. She told me to wait right there in the hallway, and quickly returned with a printed map of the neighborhood and a neatly wrapped plastic bag full of soap, as she didn't want me to have to buy soap at the laundromat. Not surprisingly, her map was very clear, and I made it to the laundromat without any mistakes. Just after I put my laundry in the wash, though, it started to rain. I hadn't thought to bring an umbrella, but just as I was contemplating the reality of a soaking-wet run home, a car pulled up to the laundromat, and out popped Reiko . . . with an umbrella! She'd taken it upon herself to devise this rescue mission to save me from impending weather doom. "After you put your laundry in the dryer, leave it there and walk back to the ryokan with the umbrella," Reiko instructed. "We don't want you to walk back with your laundry in the rain, so we will drive you back to get your laundry out of the dryer when it's finished."

I was touched. I had already accepted my fate of getting both myself and my laundry wet. But that's often how it is in Japan. Later, back at the ryokan, I told Keigo what had happened, and his face lit up with joy. "It's ichigo ichie!" he smiled.

"Ichigo ichie? I've never heard of it," I replied. "What does it mean?"

"It's a big part of omotenashi—it translates to 'one time, one meeting,' or 'once in a lifetime,'" he replied. "It means that we do our best to live in the present moment, because every-thing is impermanent. Part of that means taking our interactions very seriously, because every moment could be our last."

Later that night in my ryokan room, I Googled the concept of ichigo ichie while sipping on a Sapporo I'd grabbed from the vending machine outside my room. (Yes: Vending machines in Japan sell beer, and watching one fall down the slot is as fun as you would imagine.) While the philosophy may sound a bit like YOLO ("you only live once"), we often tend to say YOLO when we are talking about big once-in-a-lifetime activities, like sky-diving or taking that bucket-list trip. Ichigo ichie is more about appreciating the fleeting nature of everyday moments. Reiko knew I wouldn't be back again at her ryokan on that afternoon on that day on my first trip to Japan ever again, for example, so she did her best to elevate my experience.

The origins of ichigo ichie are rooted in the sadō (Japanese tea ceremony), which is one of the definitive examples of Japanese omotenashi. The tea ceremony, also referred to as the "way of tea," is an elaborate and ceremonial ritual in which Japanese tea masters prepare and present matcha (powdered green tea) to guests. Ichigo ichie first came into the picture back in the six-teenth century, when legendary tea master and Zen Buddhist Sen no Rikyū coined the term to indicate that both the host and the guest of the tea ceremony must recognize that this is a one-time, one-meeting moment, never to be replicated again. Sen no Rikyū's apprentice, Yamanoue Sōji, eventually wrote a book chronicling his master's wise teachings, in which he instructed teahouse guests to give great respect to their hosts by treating the sadō like it was the only time it could or would ever happen again in their lifetime. Even if the exact same group comes together at a later point, the logic goes, the experience will still be different. That exact moment in time is utterly unique and can never be replicated.

Today, that tea philosophy has gone far beyond the tatami mats and (quite literally) seeped its way into everyday life. Keigo told me that it's even his main wellness mantra. "I know that you're writing a book on wellness, and to me, wellness is ichigo ichie," he explained while we were hiking one afternoon. "In Buddhist philosophy, one of the core teachings is that all moments are transient and everything is impermanent. This means that you should give value to every moment in your life, especially to all of the time that you spend together with everyone you meet, because it could be your last. Living this way helps me stay present in the moment and appreciate each new day."

I spent the rest of my time in Japan alternating between hiking, soaking, eating too much food, and drinking too much sake and vending-machine beer. The Japanese have a saying, "hara hachi-bun-me ni isha irazu," which translates to "filling four-fifths of your stomach keeps the doctor away," but I don't think that it applies to travelers experiencing the joys of kaiseki for the first time.

Nor does it apply to travelers experiencing the pure joys of those ubiquitous Japanese 7-Elevens. Though the chain is in multiple countries around the world, it's owned by a company based in Tokyo, and I found its Japanese outposts to be far superior to the ones in the States. They sell delicious pre-packaged lunches, like egg salad sandwiches and onigiri (rice balls), plus a huge assortment of fun, surprising snacks (think barbecued squid rice crackers) that make strolling their aisles a guidebook-recommended activity. And they're everywhere, even considered part of the national infrastructure. In many of the quiet rural villages I stayed at along the Kumano Kodo, the ryokans and the 7-Elevens were some of the only places to get food—true sustenance oases in otherwise remote lands.

By the time I got back to New York, I was craving the 7 Eleven rice balls I'd come to love. But on a deeper level, I was also craving the feeling of presence I'd experienced in Japan. I was having a hard time re-creating that spirit in my urban life in Brooklyn, away from the ryokans and Keigo's infectious ichigo ichie essence. And so, inspired by my time with Michael, the urban Rastafari, I decided to seek out some urban tea masters in New York. How did they manage to preserve that feeling of presence and patience in a fast-paced life that can so easily whirl right on by?

I FOUND MY ANSWER AT NYC WASHITSU, A TEA-HOUSE IN UNION SQUARE SMACK DAB IN THE MIDDLE OF MANHATTAN.

Founded in 2012, Washitsu is both a school for the traditional tea ceremony and a peaceful event space where New Yorkers can gather to learn about Japanese culture. The owner, Stephen Globus, an American businessman who's spent lots of time in Japan throughout his career, originally created the space because he missed the tatami room he'd come to love at his friend's apartment in Tokyo. He hired a Japanese carpenter to transform his space, and soon enough, Japanese tea masters in New York began to ask him if they could hold traditional tea ceremonies there. One thing led to another, and now the room is a full-on tea ceremony school, with two traditional tea masters who run the show.

One of the school's tea ceremony instructors, Keiko Kitazawa Koch, invited me to the house for a traditional tea ceremony and a chat about how to keep the tea philosophies going in day-to-day life. When I arrived at Washitsu a few days later, I was instantly transported back to Japan. There was a tatami mat outside the door (shoes off, I knew), and the woodsy smell, though far away from those mountainside ryokans, still reminded me that nature exists in the world. Keiko—who moved to New York from Nara, the original capital of Japan before Tokyo, when she was twenty-seven—met me at the door in a dark blue kimono. She had one for me in her hand, too.

"I didn't actually wear a kimono in Japan, only yukatas," I told her as she wrapped mine on top of my clothes. (We didn't do a fully traditional wrap, which generally takes about half an hour.)

"Yes, kimonos are only for special occasions," she replied, "and this is a special occasion."

Traditional tea ceremonies can last up to four hours, depending on how many people are there. Everything that happens during one is a ritual, from the way the tea masters cleanse the objects, to the way they place the tea utensils in front of their guests, to the way they scoop the tea into the cup. In keeping with the Japanese tradition of ikebana, the art of flower arrangement, there is even a ritual around creating a floral display for the tea ceremony, known as chabana. Ours began

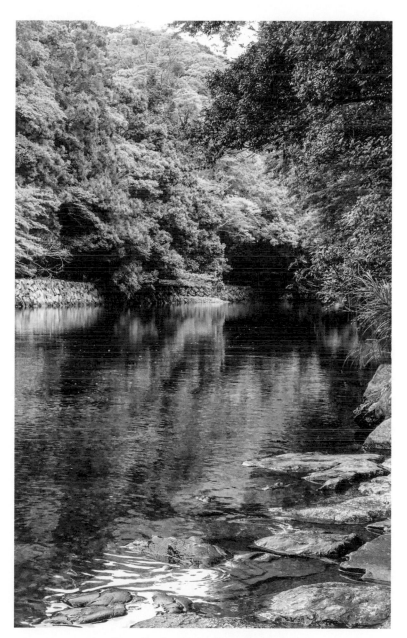

**Ise Jingu: My time in the Manhattan teahouse
took me back to serene places like this.**

when Keiko led me into the main room, which was lined with tatami mats in place of furniture. We sat on the floor next to a sunken fireplace with a black tea kettle inside. Keiko had also hung a special calligraphic scroll on the wall just for me, which is another way that Japanese tea masters honor their guests. They often spend hours—days, even—thinking about the right scroll to hang that will suit their guests' particular tastes. The scroll Keiko hung was called *Shofu Jin Gai No Kokoro* 松風塵外心. Though the original meaning translates to "the sound of the wind blowing through pine trees," *shofu* refers to the sound of boiling kiln water in the world of tea. "It means, at the time of tea, don't get distracted by the stupidity of the world—just listen to the sound of shofu and concentrate on making tea," Keiko told me. "People who live in a big city like New York are very busy. However, just this moment, forget all your stress and just listen to the shofu and relax."

I watched as Keiko brought in all of the utensils she would use to prepare my tea (a whisk, a frother, gorgeous dark blue ceramic cups) and placed them next to the sunken fireplace. Then she went about the preparations, whisking and pouring and stirring the matcha in a gentle, intentional manner. I was transfixed. "Every movement has meaning," she explained as she swirled the powdered tea around in a ceramic bowl, creating bubbles of bright green froth. "People tend to think that all Japanese people know how to do tea ceremonies, but that's not true—you have to learn each movement." After joining her first tea ceremony when she was just eight years old back in Nara, Keiko studied the "way of tea" throughout her childhood,

The Seven Rules of the Japanese Tea Ceremony,
According to Sen no Rikyū

1. Make a satisfying bowl of tea.

2. Lay the charcoal so that the water boils efficiently.

3. Provide a sense of coolness in the summer
and warmth in the winter.

4. Arrange the flowers as though they were in a field.

5. Be ready ahead of time.

6. Be prepared in case it should rain.

7. Act with utmost consideration toward your guests.

but began to dip her toe into sports and dance in her twenties. Eventually, she moved to New York to attend art school, but once she arrived, she slowly began to realize that her heart had always been with tea. "I came here to be an artist, but I can say that this is art," she explained with a smile.

Like the matcha I'd had back in Japan, the tea was bitter and pungent and a little bit earthy, an acquired taste I'd come to associate with the smell of sulfur and fresh cedar trees. But Keiko's care and devotion appealed to me even more than the flavor of travel nostalgia. I had never seen someone go to such intricate, concentrated lengths to prepare one cup of tea.

"The ritual of the tea ceremony is very valuable to me because it helps me remember that this moment never comes back," she told me in true ichigo ichie style. "If I met you at another time, it would be different. The seasons would be different; you would be different. Making this tea during this ceremony is my way of remembering that all we have is now."

"That's especially helpful in this busy city, when we're constantly operating in overdrive," I said.

"Yes," she nodded. "All we have is this moment."

After we wrapped up, Keiko bowed from the door to signify that our gathering was over. On the crowded subway back to my apartment, all too aware of the sweaty people packed in right beside me, I thought about how I'd lost myself for a minute there in the tea room. Watching Keiko prepare everything had put me in a trance. And I realized then that that's what I'd come to love most about the entire "way of tea" philosophy: It's about purposefully seeking out those moments where you're so in it, so focused on the now, that you aren't even thinking about anything else.

Shigenori Nagatomo, PhD, a professor of philosophy and East Asian Buddhism at Temple University, told me later that this idea—the art of being present—is ultimately about learning to embrace the Buddhist concept of time. "Buddhists believe that you cannot separate yourself from time, because you *are* time. Time is not something that happens to you. You and time go together. You *live* time. And so, when you apply that idea to ichigo ichie, it means that you start to ask yourself a question: What would be the best way to live that time? Will you ride the rhythm? Will you ride the waves of time? If you are time, then the best way to live it is to ride it well."

Professor Nagatomo believes that riding the waves of time well also means accepting the Buddhist idea that life is playing out right before our eyes—and we have to try to see things in real time, as they really are. "Many people often daydream," he points out, "thinking that there is something better other than where you are. But the whole idea in Buddhism is that an 'ultimate reality' is unfolding right before your eyes, right where you are, all of the time—so you want to fully engage yourself in that. Reality is not somewhere far beyond. It is right here, right where you are, so you do not want to miss it or fiddle with it."

That's why the tea masters like Keiko perform all of the elaborate rituals during the tea ceremony: It's a way to get outside of themselves and fully engage with the present moment. After all, if everything is impermanent, and time is fleeting, and life is transient, shouldn't we all just be chasing moments that free us, chasing moments that are so wonderful, so unique, they make us forget ourselves and get out of our own heads? "Most people are so caught up with themselves and don't know how to forget themselves—but ichigo ichie is the art of self-forgetting," Professor Nagatomo concluded. "Of course you have to attend to the important things in your life, but for all other times, the best way to forget yourself is to fully engage with the ultimate reality that's playing out right in front of you, whatever that may be."

Live in the Moment...

WHEREVER YOU ARE

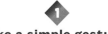

Make a simple gesture.

Next time you get together with someone, bring something meaningful that makes them happy, like their favorite flower or a book they can borrow. Their joy will increase your happiness, too.

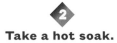

Take a hot soak.

Japanese men and women have been practicing the art of the self-care bath for more than three thousand years. The only requirement for the Japanese-inspired way is to make it an intentional and consistent part of your routine. Grab some muscle-soothing Epsom salt, draw yourself a bath, and take the moment to unwind and just be.

Master a new skill.

Quick and easy shortcuts have risen to fame in our busy society—who has the time to do anything with lots of steps? But one way to forget yourself is to get involved in something intricate, not so much for the outcome but for the process. The Japanese do this with matcha ceremonies and kaiseki dinners, but the practice can easily be applied to baking an intricate cake or knitting a sweater.

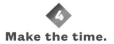

Make the time.

It can be tempting to blow people off when you're busy or in a rush. But ichigo ichie teaches us to honor those fleeting moments. Thanks to Reiko's one-time-one-meeting philosophy, that laundry experience became a highlight of my time in Japan. The next time your coworker wants to chat, or a stranger looks like they could use some help with their bags, go for it. There is only now.

Bring the outdoors inside.

My favorite part about the ryokans was the tatami mats. Smelling them helped me feel so peaceful and present when I was indoors—they were a constant and pleasant reminder that nature was just outside my window. To get the effect, bring the natural aroma of nature inside, whether that's by sprinkling cedar sachets throughout the rooms in your house, or even getting your own tatami mat.

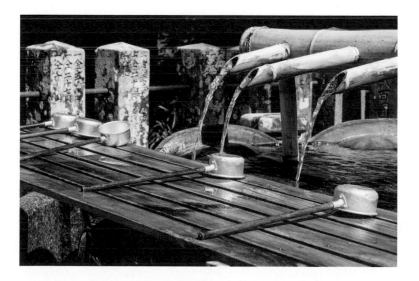

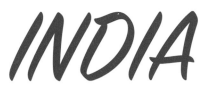

INDIA

Make It

PERSONAL

with

AYURVEDA

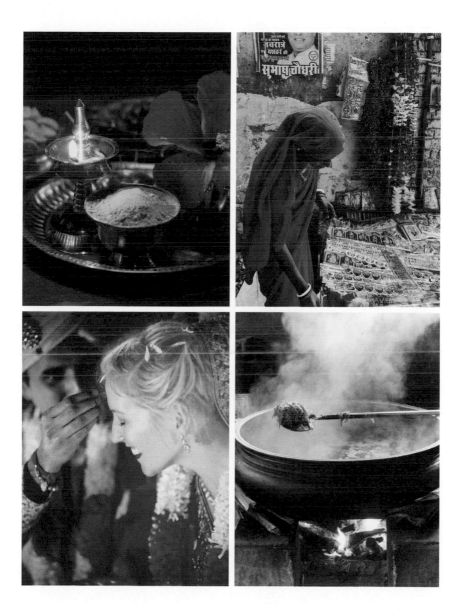

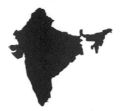

WOULD YOU LIKE coconut oil, mustard oil, or almond oil?" an older Indian man asked me after I'd gotten settled in my chair.

"Hmm . . . coconut oil!" I replied, as if I had been answering that question my whole life.

I definitely hadn't.

Although it may sound like I was sitting down at a restaurant or a bar, casually choosing a salad dressing, I was actually in a hair salon in New Delhi with Rahul, who was still my boyfriend back then, not yet my husband. In a wild leap of faith, we'd decided to travel to his home country together just three months after we met on a camping trip and started dating. There were some extenuating circumstances involved in the matter: I'd gotten a travel-writing assignment in Australia, and he had a friend's wedding to go to in Delhi at the exact time I'd be flying home from Down Under. We came up with an idea: *What if I stopped by India on my way back to New York*? I could meet his parents, see where he grew up, and attend my first Indian wedding. As a freelance travel journalist, I could write about it, too. We knew it was a little quick to dive into a meet-the-parents situation so soon after we started dating, but so what? We were falling in love and both very much fly-by-the-seat-of-your-pants people. The timing seemed too perfect, too fateful, to ignore— so we just went for it. And that's how I found myself in a salon chair in New Delhi with my head drenched in coconut oil, smelling like the beach, as my stylist kneaded his hands into my scalp and drops of oil dripped onto the towel he'd placed on my shoulders.

"That was absolutely incredible," I sighed to Rahul once we'd left the salon and were heading back to his house to put on our wedding gear (a saree for me, my first; a sherwani—a knee-length dress-up coat—for him). He'd told me that we were going to get oil head massages before his friend's wedding—a longtime pre-event ritual of his—but I had no idea *just* how much I would love the tradition until I experienced it for myself. And to top it all off, my hair was the shiniest it had been in a long time.

"Oh yeah, oil head massages are the best," he nodded. "They're super popular all around India, and they're originally rooted in Ayurveda. My mom really loves them too. You should talk to her about Ayurveda when we get home—she's really into it and I'm sure she would be so happy to tell you more about it if you're interested."

Defined as the traditional, natural medical science of life in India, Ayurveda is a huge part of Indian culture. I'd heard about it here and there, but I hadn't paid much attention to it until that head massage piqued my curiosity. Once we got home, I asked Rahul's mom, Neelam, to fill me in on the science, and when we got back from the wedding much later that night, I found a stack

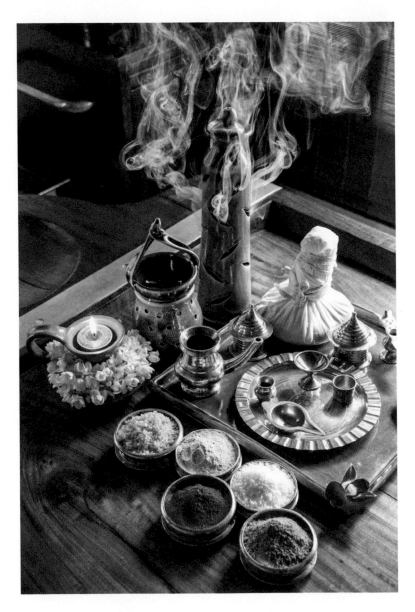

Kerala: Ayurveda uses a variety of treatments to cultivate well-being.

of her Ayurvedic books and beauty products she'd gathered from around the house waiting for me on the living room table.

"Your mom is so sweet," I whispered to Rahul, hoping not to wake anyone up. "Obviously I am about to go all in on Ayurveda now—you know this, right?"

"Of course," he replied. Even though we'd only been together for three months, he already knew that when I discover something I like, my curiosity takes over. I will read all of the articles and soak it all in until there is nothing left to soak. When we got back to the States after that inaugural trip, Rahul gave me my first Ayurveda book—*Ayurveda: The Science of Self Healing*—as I hadn't wanted to take it from his mom's collection. And my journey had officially begun.

AS YOU PROBABLY GUESSED, AYURVEDA IS ABOUT MUCH MORE THAN MAKING YOUR HAIR SHINE LIKE A FRESHLY IRONED SILK SHIRT.

Commonly referred to as the "sister science" to yoga, this ancient and complex Hindu medical healing and prevention system originated in India more than five thousand years ago. Originally passed down as an oral tradition, Ayurveda was first recorded in Sanskrit in four sacred texts known as the Vedas. The word *Ayurveda* itself, in fact, is a combination of two Sanskrit words: *ayur* (life) and *veda* (study). Translated, it quite literally means "the knowledge or study of life." Ayurveda is the blend of your soul (atma), your mind (mamas), your body (sharira), and your senses (indriyas). Generally speaking, most sciences in the Western world only focus on your mind, body, and soul, but many Ayurvedic experts

Your Natural Disposition, According to Your Dosha

While all people are made up of all three doshas, the ancient Ayurvedic texts asserted that most people generally have one dominant dosha in particular. Some people are also dual doshic, which means they have a little bit more of two doshas than the third. It's quite rare to find someone who is tridoshic, meaning their constitutions are made up of an equal amount of all three doshas. Here's a brief breakdown of what each dosha looks like.

Vata dosha (air and space)

WHEN IN BALANCE:
Physically, vata types are often thinner and lighter than the other doshas, as they don't hold a lot of Earthy elements. They may have irregular appetites and dry skin or hair, and they move quickly and frequently. Mentally, vatas tend to be highly creative, artsy, and a bit spacey. They are generally very outgoing and social, and make big life decisions on a whim. They often love to travel, they have tons of ideas, and they're very adaptable to change.

WHEN OUT OF BALANCE:
A vata imbalance is linked to eighty conditions, including pain, anxiety, and insomnia. An out-of-balance vata may lose weight and have more constipation, gas, and bloating. They may also feel overly scattered and filled with worry and fear.

Pitta dosha (fire and water)

WHEN IN BALANCE:
Physically, pitta types tend to have medium builds with strong internal fires, sensitive eyes, and red, oily skin that's prone to irritation. Mentally, pittas are likely to be ambitious, driven, and passionate. They're often analytical thinkers with excellent leadership and decision-making skills.

WHEN OUT OF BALANCE:
A pitta imbalance is linked to forty conditions, most notably inflammation. An out-of-balance pitta can become easily angry, frustrated, and judgmental.

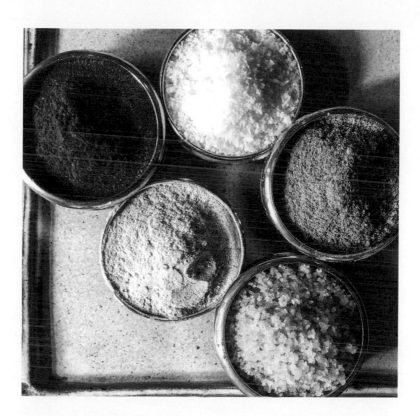

Kapha dosha (earth and water)

WHEN IN BALANCE:
Physically, kaphas tend to have strong, sturdy, compact builds, with steady digestion. Mentally, kaphas are usually very grounded, loyal, and stable. They also tend to be incredibly loving, nurturing, and empathetic.

WHEN OUT OF BALANCE:
A kapha imbalance is linked to twenty conditions, including diabetes and obesity. An out-of-balance kapha may gain weight and feel sluggish, slow, sentimental, and overly sad.

say that caring for your sense organs—your ears, eyes, nose, tongue, and skin—is actually the most important aspect of overall health, as they allow us to bring information from the outside world inward.

If you remember one thing about Ayurveda, it should be that the science looks at health individually. Ayurveda teaches its students that the five elements of life—earth, water, fire, air, and space—combine to form three different doshas, or mind-body types: vata (air and space), pitta (fire and water), and kapha (earth and water). While all humans are made up of all five elements, most of us are born with a little more of some than others, which determines our primary dosha (also known as a *prakriti,* which translates to "natural state" or "natural constitution").

According to Ayurveda, true health is when we are in perfect balance, having maintained the exact ratio of elements that we were born with. But the problem is that environmental factors like the seasons, the weather, travel, lifestyle choices, and our diets can easily throw our doshas out of whack, which is what causes distress and, eventually, disease. The whole science of Ayurveda, then, is to acknowledge that fragility and do what we can to bring our doshas back into balance. In its most simple terms, Ayurveda is all about the dedication to getting back to square one. Back to equilibrium. Think of it like a seesaw: While it's so easy to go all the way up and all the way down, Ayurveda encourages us to hang out right in the middle, so the seesaw is perfectly straight.

In India, Nepal, and other Eastern countries, Ayurveda is considered a prestigious medicine. While we tend to categorize Ayurvedic practitioners as alternative thinkers in the US, they're right up there with regular doctors in India. Their degree—a Bachelor of Ayurvedic Medicine and Surgery (BAMS)—requires five and a half years of schooling. Some of the more complex medical treatments that Ayurvedic practitioners learn during this time—like rasashastra, the therapeutic use of minerals and metals, and various steps of Panchakarma, an elaborate multi-step cleanse based on ancient purification techniques—aren't even legal to practice in full in the United States due to FDA regulations.

That said, according to India's most recent National Family Health Survey, a large-scale survey conducted in a sample of households throughout India, about 99 percent of Indians go to a doctor who practices allopathic medicine—also referred to as Western medicine—when they are sick. But Rahul and some experts I spoke with say these ancient Ayurvedic philoso-phies and recommendations are so ingrained in Indian culture that most households incorporate them into their daily routines without even thinking about it. "A lot of Indian mothers like my mom are so familiar with Ayurvedic remedies, they don't even call them Ayurvedic," Rahul told me. "They'll just say some-thing like, 'Oh, you have a cold? Take this milk with this herb' or something like that."

THE MORE I READ ABOUT AYURVEDA OVER THE YEARS, THE MORE I REALIZED HOW RELEVANT IT STILL IS TODAY. And that's why, when it came time to decide where to go for this book, I knew I had to include the southern Indian state of Kerala—the land of Ayurveda—in the mix.

On a personal level, I thought that going all in on Ayurveda could potentially help heal my troublesome skin. I'd been struggling with cystic, adult-onset acne since I graduated from college, and I hadn't had much luck with doctors. I'd taken two different oral antibiotics for eight years in a row, but they hadn't helped clear up my face. I was constantly broken out throughout my twenties, especially around my period, when I would inevitably get a cystic pimple so deep and painful that I often cancelled dates and bailed on parties and work events because I was too humiliated to be seen in such a state. And I also felt ashamed that I was writing and pitching all sorts of articles about female empowerment and loving and owning your body when I didn't love my own. I was embarrassed—and then embarrassed by my embarrassment. Was I really so vain that I couldn't get over this?

In perhaps one of the most beautiful moments of my life, my skin was at its absolute worst when I met Rahul on that fateful camping trip. I'd started a third medicine that often makes your skin worse when you begin taking it—but for the first time in a long time, I didn't run away when we started chatting. Rahul didn't stare at my irritated skin (trust me, I can tell when someone is looking), and ever since then, he's taken it upon himself to help me through my struggles with gentleness and grace. During a particularly brutal breakout, he suggested that I try to get off all of the skin medicines entirely—because they clearly weren't working. "Maybe Ayurveda or something similarly natural can help," he said.

After he brought up the possibility of going off my medications, I started to wonder: Why *had* I continued to take the drugs for so many years? Why *hadn't* I looked for a more natural solution like Ayurveda? I began to realize that, like so many of my fellow Americans, I'd been mindlessly taking prescriptions my doctor had given me without pausing to consider the root cause of my problem to determine a more personalized approach. I didn't have the patience to experiment with more-natural solutions that may have worked best for me; I wanted a quick fix.

Meanwhile, those popular pharmaceutical options often came with commercials showing someone frolicking in a field of sunflowers, only to end with long, fast-talking monologues about all of the potential side effects. Of course, there is a time and a place for pharmaceutical drugs, but it is worth noting that

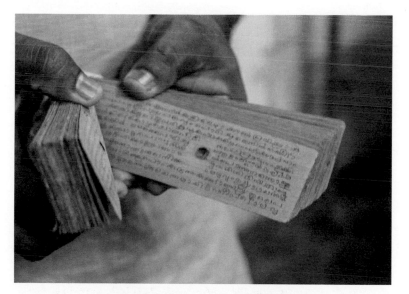

Kerala: Some of the ancient Ayurvedic texts,
which now live at the Ayurveda Museum.

the United States and New Zealand are the only countries in the entire world where direct-to-consumer advertising of prescription drugs is even *legal*. I'd spent years thinking that they were the only option because my dermatologist prescribed them to me and that was that. But the more I read about Ayurveda, the more I became open to the possibility that there was another way to heal.

During this skin revelation of mine, I'd also started to notice another more universal reason that personalized healthcare could be particularly relevant today: Our cultural definition of well-being in America was becoming increasingly homogenous. During my time working at the wellness magazine, I saw firsthand just how much "wellness" had started to take off. The word itself had become synonymous with kale salad, and then barre class, and then women clad in leggings carrying tote bags that say "but first, coffee." It was such a narrow and non-inclusive definition of well-being.

I knew, of course, that following the same diet and fitness trends is nothing entirely new. Americans have been doing this for decades, from embracing the hula hoop trend in the 1950s to Jazzercise in the 1970s to indoor Spinning in the 1990s to the Zumba craze in the early 2000s. Same with food: We've collectively abandoned carbs and then embraced them, kicked fat to the curb and then taken it back, really leaned into the whole cottage cheese thing only to replace it a few years later with all avocado everything. But the difference between now and then is that social media has amplified everything, so those trends have started to reach even more people, and at a faster rate. Instead of listening to what our own body wants and needs, as Ayurveda teaches, many of us choose instead to listen to what the algorithm wants and needs: spectacle food and cool-looking workouts. And that collective quest for universally 'gram-worthy content leaves little room for the Ayurvedic philosophy that everyone shouldn't be going after the same things at all.

Since I'd started dabbling in Ayurvedic knowledge about five years ago, trying out a few natural skin remedies and routines here and there, I'd returned to India six other times with Rahul. We'd traveled all over the country, from the fresh-air mountain mecca that is the Himalayas to the palace-filled states in Rajasthan to the star-studded beaches of Goa to the Bollywood center of Mumbai. I'd seen countless Ayurvedic centers in all of those places, and eaten countless Ayurvedic dishes on countless menus scattered throughout the country. But Kerala, I knew, was where you went when you wanted to *know* Ayurveda, to learn how to be so dialed into Ayurveda that you were able to continue its teachings at home. And I wanted to be on that level.

For someone who'd already traveled to India six times in five years, though, I was surprisingly nervous to travel to Kerala for my seventh trip—because I was going to be in India without Rahul. While he wanted to come to Kerala with me, he couldn't take enough time off work that month to come. I obviously love solo traveling, but the thought of solo traveling in *India* was different. How could I be in India without the man who has defined my India experience? It's well documented that India is one of the most difficult places to travel as a Westerner, but the truth is that when I'm with Rahul, my experience is pretty deluxe. Of course Rahul is my life partner, but in India, he's also my translator who makes it easy to get around in a rickshaw, and my tour guide who tells me exactly what we're looking at as we go by, and my foodie who makes sure we eat only the most delicious dishes—and avoid traveler's dysentery. What would India be without all of those built-in luxuries? Perhaps more important, would I even enjoy India as much as I have in the past? To me, India *is* Rahul, so I wondered: *Do I love India because I love Rahul, or would I love India on its own no matter what?*

I was still grappling with these questions when I touched down in Kochi, the capital of Kerala, and the thick, tropical air wrapped around me like a sticky bun as soon as I stepped off the plane. I love tropical atmospheres, and at around 10 degrees north—the equivalent of Costa Rica, for context—Kerala is a dream. Although the origin of the word *Kerala* is debatable, one prominent theory says that it's derived from the Malayalam (Kerala's local language) words *kera* (coconut) and *alam* (land), meaning it translates to "The Land of Coconut Trees." Located on the southwest coast of India, right on the Arabian Sea, the state is known for its stunning white-sand beaches and its backwaters, which is a weirdly unpoetic name for its network of serene canals, lagoons, lakes, and rivers that lie parallel to the sea. Parts of Kerala have even been referred to as the "Venice of the East," and have also been compared to the American bayous.

"Annie?" my driver asked me when he saw me looking at the sign he was holding outside of baggage claim.

I nodded yes as I wiped a bunch of sweat from my already drenched face. My phone said it was only 80°F, but that didn't factor in the muggy humidity. "Let's get into the car and blast the A/C!" I told him.

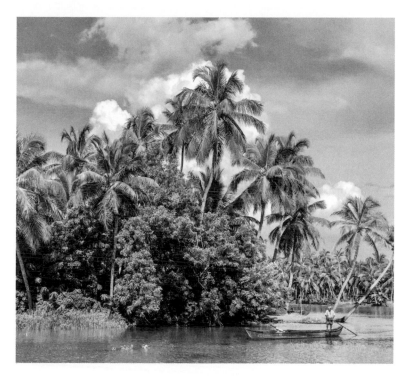

Kerala: The famous backwaters look like a tropical postcard.

Weeks before my trip, I'd made a reservation for a seven-day Ayurvedic immersion program at the Nattika Beach Ayurveda Hospital and Resort in Thrissur, Kerala, about two hours south of Kochi. Think of the *hospital* label like the Michelin star of Ayurvedic centers: If you see the word in the title, you know it's going to be legit. It's the highest accreditation for an Ayurvedic retreat center in India, an honorable title given by the central government that means the center has an exceptionally intelligent and qualified staff of doctors, clean and up-to-date treatment rooms, quality food, and programming designed to help you both heal from and prevent illness. In the States, we often wait until we are sick to go to a doctor. But Ayurvedic philosophy means being proactive and preventative about health. The ancient take is: Why wait until you're sick when you can do everything you can now to stay well?

I booked Nattika because it had that hospital street cred, but still sounded like a lovely spot to get into a spiritual zone, with fifty-two villas set among 16 acres of coconut groves, plus a cafeteria where you eat all your meals, a yoga hut, and the hospital itself, which is packed with certified Ayurvedic doctors and therapists whose job is to guide you through a regimented program. To be clear, it's not the only place like this in Kerala; it's just the one that I happened to choose. One joint report from the nonprofit association Confederation of Indian Industry and PricewaterhouseCoopers—which was first disclosed at the Global Ayurveda Summit in Kochi—found that the southern state has 1,400 Ayurveda-associated industries, with a total profit of $37 million in 2016. And experts predict that with the growing focus on health and well-being around the world, Kerala is going to become much more popular. It was the first state in the country to launch a responsible tourism initiative, but it's already showing signs of overtourism.

The drive through Kerala, from the airport in Kochi to Nattika in Thrissur, was colorful in all senses of the word. We passed women walking on the street in gorgeously bold sarees. We passed an array of two-story houses in an explosion of tropical tones, with giant coconut palms swaying in the wind. Fuchsia bougainvillea clung to the walls of the houses like a statement necklace, adding that quintessential "pop of color" magazine editors have preached about for years. We even passed a couple of big, hippie-style busses painted in bright yellows and blues that looked like they were straight out of a Ken Kesey novel. Throughout this entire feast for the eyes, I kept thinking: *Is this really India?* To me, India was the hazy smog of Delhi that enveloped the sun, casting a subtle golden haze over the city that never really clears up. It was the sparkly, crown-jewel palaces of Rajasthan that transported me to the medieval era, and the little mountain towns in the Himalayas where the only thing fresher than the air was the morning parathas. The farthest south I'd been was Goa, so Kerala was new to me. While I did miss Rahul, I was also so far removed from his India, my India, *our* India, that it hardly even felt like I was there without him. I was in an India of my own.

"THE BODY IS A UNION OF ABOUT FIFTY TRILLION CELLS DESIRING TO BE TOGETHER AND TO WORK TOGETHER AND TO LIVE IN HARMONY. BUT USUALLY, MAYBE ABOUT 10 PERCENT OF THOSE CELLS WILL BECOME A BIT NAUGHTY AND THEY WILL START DOING SOMETHING REALLY SILLY."

My Ayurvedic practitioner at Nattika, Dr. Hema K.P., told me about this "silliness" with a very straight face, in a matter-of-fact tone, on my first day at the hospital. I'd only been there for about an hour—just long enough to settle into my airy, ceramic-tiled hut before making my way to my initial consultation—and I was already learning new ways of thinking.

"And then the other 90 percent will try to tell them, *come on, behave yourself*," she continued. I let out a little laugh then, and Dr. Hema, a woman on the shorter side with a gentle and firm manner, looked at me super seriously: "This is absolutely what is happening. Ayurveda is about having concern for both the healthy 90 percent and the naughty 10 percent—you need to keep them in balance."

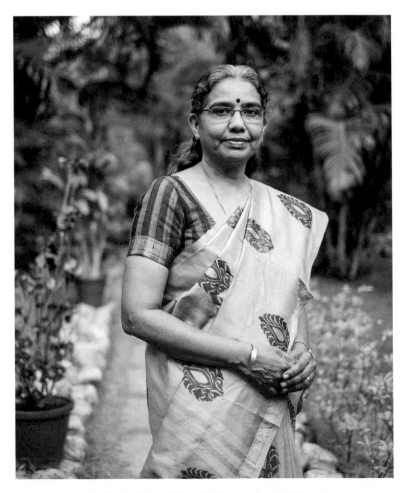

Kerala: Dr. Hema K.P., chief Ayurveda physician at Nattika and my knowledgeable Ayurveda guide.

Sitting there listening to Dr. Hema speak for the first time, my initial knee-jerk reaction, one cultivated through years of science-backed health reporting at national publications in New York, was to question her logic. What did that even mean, keeping naughty cells in balance? Were there studies about that? But the more time I spent with her, the more I realized that *I* was the one whose logic could use an upgrade. And eventually, in the war between my health-editor brain ("give me proof!") and my travel-editor brain ("give me an open mind!"), my travel brain won.

Look: There are a couple of scientific studies that suggest that Ayurvedic philosophies and treatments may reduce pain, and a few promising bits of research that prove that curcumin— the most active compound in turmeric, one of Ayurveda's most popular herbs—may help fight inflammation. But most of them are small or poorly executed or only done in a laboratory rather than a clinical trial, meaning they are not to be fully trusted by Western medical standards. The more time I spent at Nattika, though, the more I started to realize that I shouldn't be looking to those studies for proof in the first place. This is a life science that has been around for millennia helping Indians heal for more than five thousand years. Shouldn't that be enough?

Viewing Ayurveda's health lessons through an American lens calls for a shift in thinking and a reminder that it's not always possible to apply our Western thinking to Eastern ways. It was on me, I realized, to learn about how Ayurveda works in India with an open mind. And it was on me to take away lessons that broaden my horizons, lessons that are not necessarily steeped in proof in the way I was trained to think of proof, but can be valuable and effective and spiritual nonetheless. These are the three philosophies I found to be the most useful and applicable to our modern times:

You don't always get to choose what's best for your body. In Ayurveda, your body chooses for you.

American spas may give you a list of treatments they offer and ask you to select what you want and when you want it. At Ayurvedic hospitals, the practitioners do the choosing for you— and their selections are based entirely on your genetic makeup. While I can only speak to my personal experience at Nattika, the process is generally the same no matter where you are: After you check in, you meet with your personalized on-site Ayurvedic practitioner to determine your dominant dosha (or doshas). Practitioners are trained to determine doshas through a combination of questions about your lifestyle (what happens to you when you're stressed out; what kind of sleeper are you; what would you consider to be your general temperament), and by reading your pulse, an ancient practice known as *nadi vijnan*. (Dr. Hema determined that I have a pitta-vata constitution, but I'm predominantly pitta.)

During this initial meeting, your practitioner also asks you what you hope to accomplish during your stay: Are you there to heal a particular ailment, or focus on overall rejuvenation? The next day and every morning after that, you meet with your practitioner again, who starts by asking how you slept and how your "toilets" (poop) were when you woke up. (Cleaning out your system every morning is a very important

Ayurvedic practice, as the ancient Ayurvedic texts asserted that good digestion leads to better health overall.) Then, your practitioner asks you how you're feeling so far that day. Unlike Western medicine, which is often more focused on the physical body, Ayurveda places equal emphasis on your emotional state—it is the balance of the mind, body, soul, and senses, after all.

The ancient practitioners understood the mind-body connection right from the start: If your mind is not well, your body is not well. Like many Americans, I was raised to believe that you only go to the doctor when something is physically wrong with you. Dr. Hema helped me unlearn this idea by giving value to all questions on her list, from "how did you sleep" (physical health) to "how are you feeling" (mental health). They're all part of the greater whole.

Food is also a big part of your stay at an Ayurvedic hospital. Once you know your dosha, you meet with an on-site nutritionist, who gives you an eating plan for breakfast, lunch, and dinner throughout your stay, all based on your current personal constitution. In the cafeteria at Nattika, each dish was labeled by dosha, which made it very easy for me to eat only pitta-balancing foods and teas and punt the rest—but man was I eyeing those kapha curries! (More on how to eat with your dosha in mind later.)

Finally, it's time for your therapists to administer whatever treatments your doctor recommended for the day. "The treatments are only decided after we assess the condition of each person and the imbalance of their doshas," Dr. Hema told me. She and I decided that my main goal while I was there was to reduce my overall inflammation in the hopes of getting clearer skin, and once she had that information, she devised a treatment plan just for me—a true no-substitutions treatment plan that involved various "face baths" (what they call a facial treatment). And I was petrified. I'd gone off of all of my skin medicines at that point, and although I appreciated not being on them, I was still prone to random breakouts. One day my skin would be fine, and then it would flare up from stress or hormones or who knows what else—I've stopped trying to pinpoint the cause. But all of this angst had built up over many years and resulted in my extreme fear of putting anything on my face except gentle face wash and oil-free makeup. At our wedding, Rahul and I did haldi ceremonies, a ritual where your guests slather turmeric paste all over your clothes and your face for good luck before your ceremony, and I was fine then— so I had a feeling that I would be okay. Still, that was just one ritual, and I was signing up for seven days of face bathing here, where they'd put all sorts of stuff on my skin. What if I broke out?

My first face bath was a raw buttermilk and papaya mask that smelled like barfi, an Indian sweet made from milk, sugar, and dried fruit. Although the mixture did feel soothing on my skin, I couldn't shake the thought that I was wearing a sugary dessert on my face—and I equated sugary desserts with breakouts. But when I asked my therapist if I could swap out the buttermilk for another ingredient, I was met with a firm no. Buttermilk and papaya, I was told, were two of the most soothing ingredients for my inflamed pitta skin, and it was the best treatment for my face.

Another ingredient I was given but did not know I needed was oil. Thanks to my initial coconut-oil head massage, and to Rahul's mom Neelam, I knew that oiling (yeah, it's a verb) is a big part of Ayurveda. But I had no idea *just* how central the practice is to the whole lifestyle until I went to Nattika. Of the two hours of required treatments every day, most of them involved oil (though my therapists never put oil on my face, due to my sensitive skin). The benefits of slathering yourself in oil go all the way back to *Ashtanga Hridaya Sutrasthana,* one of the four ancient Ayurvedic texts. The text states that abhyanga (oil massage) should be done daily, and that it slows down aging, relieves fatigue, improves skin health, and more. Gwyneth Paltrow has gone on the record countless times to preach the benefits of oiling, and I've gotta say, after oiling for seven straight days, this is perhaps one of the few areas where I actually agree with her: We really *do* need to be oiling ourselves way more often.

Even though I'm an oiling convert now, though, my first experience was not so smooth. A traditional oil massage involves a therapist dousing you in warm, medicated oils infused with herbs that help pacify your dosha, and then rubbing it all over your body in long, sweeping motions. When I walked into the open-foyer treatment room, there were two dark wooden massage tables, a knee-high stool in the middle of the room, a couple sticks of incense burning, and a few medium-sized areca palm trees, with their narrow bamboo-like fronds swaying in the breeze. The room was mostly dark, save for the square of natural light streaming down on the floor from the open foyer, and my therapist, a shorter, older woman named Vijayakumari

(Vijay for short), smiled hello and handed me what looked like a piece of white cloth. She then instructed me to take off my clothes.

I waited for her to leave the room, as massage therapists in the US do, but she just stood there, watching me. "Oh, here?" I asked her. Having just been in the onsens in Japan, I was getting more used to nudity with strangers, but still, stripping down directly in front of her seemed a bit much. "Yes, here," she laughed.

So I went for it: I slowly took off my shirt, then my leggings, and then my sports bra, depositing them into my tote bag right in front of her. Finally, I was left standing there in my underwear, and she nodded to tell me that, yes, it was time to take that off, too. Once I was fully naked, she took the white cloth from my hand and tied it around me like a diaper, then instructed me to sit on the stool in the middle of the room—at which point she began singing a pre-massage prayer.

Have you ever had someone sing to you in the dark while you are sitting naked and upright on a wooden stool, with nothing between your butt and the cold wood but a piece of cloth? Vijay's voice was so beautiful it almost made me cry. For the next hour, we communicated primarily through body language and touch, since I don't speak Malayalam, and Vijay didn't speak much English, except for a couple phrases. She was so loving, and I could tell once she started massaging my head and then covered my whole body (minus my face) with medicated oil that she treated her Ayurvedic work very seriously.

Lying there on that dark wooden massage table, I began to feel a little guilty for how much time and energy Vijay was expending to ultimately bring me into balance and clear up my skin. Yes, I was paying for her services, but still: She was pouring her heart and soul into these treatments. She sang a *prayer* song for me before my massage! I wasn't used to doctors and therapists treating me with such TLC. I wasn't even sick! My guilt got worse after a couple more days, because the treatments got more involved and elaborate. The next day, I got another abhyanga massage, only this time there were *two* therapists, and they synchronized their strokes—which is the ultimate Kerala specialty. Another day, I got a siro dhara treatment, which is when a therapist drips heated medicated oil from a pot onto your forehead (which for me is less sensitive) in a steady rhythm for nearly an hour (*siras* means "head" and *dhara* means "continuous flow"). With each passing treatment, I felt more overwhelmed by the beauty of it all, and by the attention I was receiving each day.

After a couple days of grappling with this explosion of feelings, I called Rahul to talk it out. He pointed out that maybe it wasn't just guilt I was feeling—it also sounded like admiration. "In the US, we're not used to doctors spending so much time on us for a seemingly simple problem, especially when you're not technically sick by Western standards," he reminded me. "Of course you're paying to be there, but even when you're paying in the States, you usually have to be in a much worse state to get that much attention. Ayurvedic practitioners, on the other hand, take non-critical issues and prevention just as seriously. If someone here goes to the doctor because their back is slightly hurting, the doctor will probably just send them away to a physical therapist to get one or maybe a couple massages. But Ayurvedic doctors will turn it into a whole thing, working with you to figure out why it's hurting and give you hours of personalized treatments to fix the root of the problem—and that's something you're not as used to seeing."

"Wow, that's so true," I replied, processing what he was saying. I knew, of course, that we live in a Band-Aid nation, and are more likely to choose the quick fix over the deep dive. But experiencing the deep dive firsthand made me realize *just* how much we're losing when we go for the surface solution. What we're really losing is the ability to see ourselves whole, the ability to connect all of our internal dots. Ayurvedic practitioners are professional dot connectors. They know that rubbing oil all over my body may not clear up my acne directly, but it may help pacify my pitta, which will then nudge me back into balance, which will then make me less likely to break out in the future. They play the long game. And if ancient history is any indication, the long game usually wins.

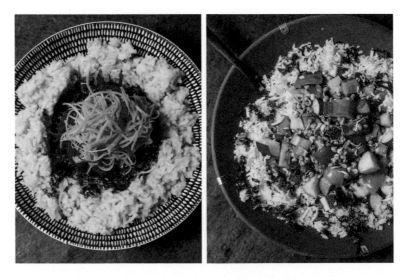

Kerala: In Ayurveda, food is (very flavorful) medicine.

It's important to eat according to your dosha.

Proper gut health is an increasingly popular topic, with more and more scientific research coming out about the link between your gut health and your mental and physical health. This is a finding Ayurvedic practitioners know all too well: They've been preaching this truth for centuries. The ancient texts said that maintaining a strong agni (digestive fire) is one of the fundamental building blocks of well-being. When your digestion is good, the texts say, your overall health is usually good. Weak digestion is usually an indicator that there are other problems at play—and potentially even more down the line.

One of the best ways to ensure that your digestion is balanced and stays on track is to eat in accordance with your dosha. "Every taste in the world has some sort of influence on our doshas, so it's very important to eat with your dosha in mind—it's the key to keeping yourself in balance," my on-site dietician, Dr. Nitha Gopalan, told me during our first meeting. She also taught me that, according to ancient Ayurvedic wisdom, cooked foods are much easier to digest than raw foods—a lesson I knew all too well. Rahul's mom often calls us after dinner to ask what we ate that night (a typical Indian mother question), and when we say salads, she'll laugh and say: "Salad is not a meal! Meals are supposed to be warm! Warm foods are better for you!"

Because of my pitta dominance, Dr. Nitha recommended that I stick with pitta-balancing foods all week, which meant no spicy or salty food whatsoever—because those would just aggravate my already hot internal fire. This was soul-crushing for me, as I love spicy and salty food, and I was in South India, of all places—known for their spicy curries! That said, although I don't have any numbers or "proof" that I was more balanced by the end of the week, I did feel great, and I didn't even miss the spicy food by the end. After I left Nattika, I spent two days at a regular hotel in Kochi, and I wasn't even tempted by the spicy South Indian curries on the menu. I just wanted to continue my natural high, so I ate mostly simple foods like dal (lentils).

There are entire books written on what to eat for your dosha, and it's nearly impossible to cover such a broad scope in one chapter, but here's a general overview, according to Dr. Nitha.

Vata dosha

BEST FOODS AND SPICES: warm, nutritious dishes that border on the heavy side (soups, stews, and warm milky drinks); legumes and root vegetables; tropical fruits (pineapples, mangos, bananas, avocados, and ripe oranges); dairy (butter, buttermilk, soft cheese, ghee, and milk); soothing spices (black pepper, ginger, cumin, garlic, cardamom, mustard, fenugreek)

FOODS TO AVOID/REDUCE: dry food products (chips and crackers); raw vegetables; cool drinks and ice cream; bitter foods

Pitta dosha

BEST FOODS AND SPICES: cooling foods (leafy vegetables and cold grains); dairy (milk, butter, and ghee); sweet and ripe fruits (mango, melon, apple, banana, and dates); cooling spices (coriander, cumin, cardamom, mint, saffron, and cloves)

FOODS TO AVOID/REDUCE: red meat and other meat-based products; hot, sour, and spicy foods and spices (black pepper and chile)

Kapha dosha

BEST FOODS AND SPICES: baked or grilled proteins and vegetables; grains (barley, millet, and oats); low-fat milk products (goat cheese and pure traditional buttermilk); nearly all spices

FOODS TO AVOID/REDUCE: Any food that's too cold, too fatty, or too oily; bread, sweets, and most processed junk foods

---

Aside from eating with your dosha in mind, Ayurveda also emphasizes the importance of eating seasonally, as the weather can quickly throw you out of balance as well. Rather than dividing the year into the four typical seasons, Ayurveda divides them by dosha:

Vata season (late fall to early winter)
Pitta season (late spring to early fall)
Kapha season (from the darkest part of winter into spring)

While eating for your dosha should be your primary focus, consider the seasonal aspect if you still feel unbalanced. It's not uncommon for pittas to feel a kapha imbalance during kapha season, for example.

Ayurvedic Staples to Keep in Your Home

While the benefits of coconut oil, cinnamon, and turmeric have already made their way into the American wellness zeitgeist, there are many Ayurvedic ingredients that deserve equal attention. Here are some that are used for both cooking and beauty remedies, plus their health benefits according to the Ayurvedic texts. All of the herbs and spices listed below are tridoshic—meaning they're great for all three doshas—and you can find them at the grocery store, online, or at your local Indian specialty store.

HERBS AND SPICES FOR COOKING	HOW AND WHY TO USE THEM
Cardamom (pods or powder)	This sweet and warming spice is an excellent digestive and helpful for bloating. I like it best in chai, and in my oatmeal.
Cumin (seeds or powder)	It speeds up digestion and soothes inflammation. Rahul's mom starts every dish she makes by sautéing cumin and coriander seeds in ghee—an Indian cooking trifecta.
Coriander (seeds or powder)	This cooling spice aids digestion and inflammation. Try coriander water—just boil 1 teaspoon of coriander seeds in a cup of water, and strain.
Fennel seeds	Eat them after a meal to help digestion and freshen the breath (they taste like licorice). Sauté them in ghee, or add them to baked goods and rice puddings.
Brahmi leaves	Primarily known as a memory booster, they calm your nerves, too. Sauté the leaves in stir-fries, and add them to dal or chutneys.

HERBS AND SPICES FOR COOKING	HOW AND WHY TO USE THEM
Asafoetida (hing) powder	This plant has a strong smell, a bit like sulfur, but the scent dissolves after cooking and the spice ultimately tastes like leeks. Best in bean and lentil dishes, it aids digestion, curbs inflammation, and, for women, helps soothe period cramps.
Ashwagandha powder or supplements	This is an adaptogen, meaning it helps the body fight stress and anxiety. Most people take it as a supplement or in powdered form rather than cooking with it. (Real talk, it doesn't taste good in food. Try drinking it with honey, milk, and other sweet additions like dates and maple syrup instead.)

FACE BATH INGREDIENTS	HOW AND WHY TO USE THEM
Besan flour (chickpea flour)	A staple base ingredient in face baths, it's especially soothing for anti-acne treatments.
Papaya	The pulp is an Ayurvedic gold mine. It helps nourish and exfoliate regular skin and even clear up inflamed skin.
Organic rosewater	It helps heal skin and reduce inflammation.
Raw buttermilk	This fermented milk (used to make the famously tangy Indian drink lassi) has cooling properties that help reduce redness and irritation.
Triphala powder	Rich in antioxidants, it helps soothe inflammation.

**Master the art of routine—
but do it for the right reason.**

One of the most defining lessons of Ayurveda is dinacharya—having a daily routine that is structured around the circadian rhythms of the Earth. The reason for having such a routine is twofold: First, participating in healthy-living maintenance tasks every day means you are less likely to fall sick down the line. And second, when you do the same thing every day, you're more likely to notice if something feels different. "It's easier to understand what has changed if you have something to compare it to, and then it's also easier to make the small changes that are needed if necessary," Dr. Hema told me.

What I loved most about dinacharya, though, was what it's *not* about: productivity. In the past couple years, Americans have developed a cultural obsession with morning routines. We celebrate successful people who wake up early and go to bed early and get it done, and we want to know how they do it so that we can do it, too. We are obsessed with people who fire off a dozen emails before going on their morning run and heading off to hustle at their Fortune 500 company. If Bill Gates eats half a grapefruit at 5:26 a.m., the logic goes, maybe we should all start to do that, too—and then maybe we can all be as successful as Bill Gates. (Unclear if Bill Gates actually eats half a grapefruit at 5:26 a.m. I made that up.)

This is, of course, foolish logic. Celebrating routines that lead to greater productivity means that we now associate routines with our output, rather than just our . . . put. When was the last time you read about an unsuccessful person who wakes up early and makes a bowl of oatmeal, only to have a boring, mediocre day afterward, where they question their life choices and send weird memes to their coworkers? Never—we want to hear about people whose early-bird tendencies set them up for success later on in the day. Failure is not on the agenda.

In Ayurveda, routine is not cloaked in the guise of productivity—routine is genuinely tied to health. Doing roughly the same thing at the same time each day helps establish balance in your constitution and keep you grounded, which ultimately promotes inner peace, discipline, happiness, and longevity. Ayurvedic practitioners favor routines not so they can do more later, but so they can take care of their well-being and notice right away if something feels off. I love that difference. There is

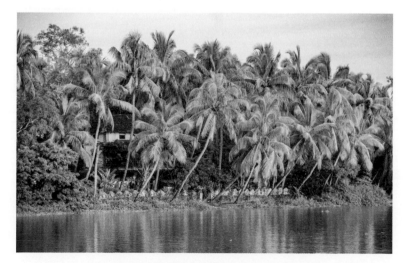

Kerala: In Ayurveda, golden-hour light means
it's time to start winding down your day.

A Dose of Dinacharya
(Daily Routine)

The following tips for how to structure your day with your health in mind come from the ancient Ayurvedic texts by way of Dr. Sreekala Santosh, Nattika's deputy chief physician. Please note: This is what an ideal Ayurvedic day looks like according to ancient wisdom. Do not feel discouraged if you can't or don't want to do all of these things! You can start wherever you want and go from there. File under "Good to know—will act accordingly."

Morning

Wake up early.
Ayurveda doesn't recommend doing so just to get more done. Early Ayurvedic texts place great importance on Brahma Mahurta, which is the auspicious time before sunrise (usually from about 4 to 6 a.m., depending on where you live and what season it is). Rising during these early-morning hours is ideal, the texts say, because it's the best time to obtain self-knowledge; there are fewer distractions from the outside world. If waking up this early is just not going to happen for you, don't worry about it. You can still do the following Ayurvedic maintenance tasks whenever they're suitable for you.

Drink a glass of warm water right after you wake up.
Add a slice of lemon if you want. Doing so helps you . . .

. . . Make time for your "toilets."
While many of us think that we need coffee to make it happen in the morning, warm water actually does the job, too.

Brush your teeth, wash your face, and wash your eyes with cool water.
Then, put a couple drops of nasya (nose) oil or powder in your nose—you can get it online. Ayurveda teaches us that the nose is the door to the brain, so cleaning it out helps improve mental clarity.

Clean your tongue with a tongue scraper.
This helps remove plaque from your tongue and strengthens your taste buds.

Gargle with unrefined sesame oil for a few minutes and then spit it out.
According to Ayurveda, this practice, called *oil pulling*, nourishes the facial nerves and muscles, and helps prevent gum disease, cavities, and bad breath. (Be sure it's raw sesame oil as opposed to toasted sesame oil, which is often used in Chinese cooking.)

Meditate for ten minutes.

Afternoon/Evening

Make lunch your biggest meal of the day.
This is when your digestion is at its strongest.

Likewise, try to have an early dinner.
Make it warm and smaller than your lunch. Large, late-night meals often cause indigestion and can rob you of your sleep.

Practice yoga asanas (the poses) and pranayama (breathing exercises).

Practice abhyanga.
Massage your whole body with oil, wait for ten minutes, and then follow it with a warm shower. This helps reduce fatigue and stress, and promotes sleep and longevity. You can use coconut oil or sesame oil, or buy a medicated oil for your dosha online.

Massage your feet and palms for five minutes just before you go to sleep.
This foot massage, known as *padabhyanga*, may help you sleep better, improve blood circulation, relieve aches and pains, and help you relax and manage depression. If you have a partner, you can do it for each other.

Try to be in bed by 10 p.m.
According to the ancient texts, this is when the laziness of kapha dominates—and when you are likely to be the most sleepy. If you stay up past ten, you may get a second wind, making it much harder to fall asleep.

so much value in opening up our minds and training ourselves to think in other ways as best as we can.

POST-KERALA, MY HAIR AND SKIN LOOKED THE BEST THEY'D EVER LOOKED.

Finally, I could use "radiant" and "my face" in the same sentence and actually not laugh at myself for doing so. I texted a glowing selfie to my friend Sophie, and she replied, "You look amazing! What did they DO to you there?"

What they *did* to me there was show me the Ayurvedic way. But I don't have the proper American "backup" to prove how much it impacted me. In that scientific context, I can't explain why the Ayurvedic way made me feel and look like the golden sky during sunset, a human equivalent of the gloaming.

There were certain fundamental elements, of course: I didn't drink alcohol for a week, which always helps your immune system get back to baseline. I likely slept better as a result of not drinking and going to bed around 8:30 p.m. (no Wi-Fi or TVs in the room will do that to you). I practiced yoga. I wrote in my journal, which always makes me feel more like me. But then there are the other, less "provable" variables: I drank pitta tea—a blend of herbs and spices including chamomile, coriander, cilantro, cardamom, saffron, fennel, licorice, peppermint, rose petals, and hibiscus—every day. I slathered myself in homemade medicated herbal-infused oils and bathed in warm milk. I ate in accordance with my dosha, which for me meant no spicy foods, no salt, and all sorts of pitta-balancing herbs, like coriander and cumin. And I leaned into the daily papaya and buttermilk face bath. I realized that, in my fear of putting anything on my face, I'd been missing out on actually *nourishing* it with ingredients that soothe my skin type. And those ingredients certainly don't require a prescription—they all come straight from the Earth.

Mostly, though, I spent time doing what's best for *me*, for *my* personal well-being. As a journalist who covers the wellness industry, I am often tasked with trying out new workouts and foods just to see what the hype is about. But while reporting on these new trends is interesting, it also means that I'm less likely to seek out something with my own personal constitution in mind. My time at Nattika changed all that. Ever since my return, I've made a conscious effort to weave Ayurvedic practices into my life. I start each day with a glass of warm water before my coffee, and give myself a chickpea flour and rosewater face bath every week or two. To tend to my emotions, I've started to write in my journal more frequently as well, and when I start to feel uneven, I cut back on the meat and the spicy food. I can't say I feel balanced all the time, but these practices do help me reel myself in before things get too dire.

In the end, that's my favorite part about practicing Ayurveda at home: It's always there for me. I will be the first to admit that I am not going to do all of the dinacharya things every day—who has the time? But it's nice to know that I can lean into Ayurveda when I feel myself swinging too far one way and I want to get back to the other side, whether that's in my mood or in my skin or in my general temperament. If there is one thing that my time in Kerala taught me, it's that we can—and should—take our health into our own hands. And those hands should probably be slathered in oil.

Stay Balanced with Ayurveda...

WHEREVER YOU ARE

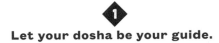

① Let your dosha be your guide.

Ayurveda teaches us that there is not a one-size-fits-all model when it comes to well-being. We are all built differently, so what's "healthy" for one person is not healthy for all. Imbalance is a constant part of living, but taking your predominant dosha into account, however loosely, can help you bring yourself back into balance.

② Consider the seasons.

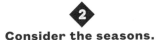

Although living by your dosha should take precedence overall, the seasons have a big impact on your internal balance as well. During kapha season, for example (late winter to early spring), you may feel more sluggish than usual—so it could be a good idea to factor light and warm kapha-balancing foods, like cooked leafy greens and grains, into your diet as well.

Put your digestion first.

Eating for your dosha is the best way to keep your agni (digestive fire) in order. Drinking warm water when you wake up, eating mostly cooked meals instead of raw foods, and making lunch your biggest meal all help, too. Try these tips . . . and then see how your "toilets" are.

Start an oiling habit.

The most memorable lesson I took away from Nattika is that oil is the crucial health ingredient we need to be using more of every day. Try all of the ways to incorporate it into your day—from oil pulling to the occasional pre-shower oil massage—and see what sticks.

Create a daily health routine.

This is a proactive way to prevent future disease—and to keep tabs on your health in the present. Start with one or two recommendations from the dinacharya list, and then add more as you see fit.

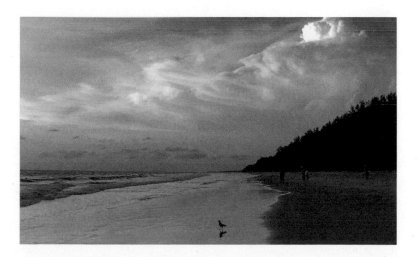

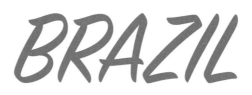

BRAZIL

EMBRACE

Your

COMMUNITY

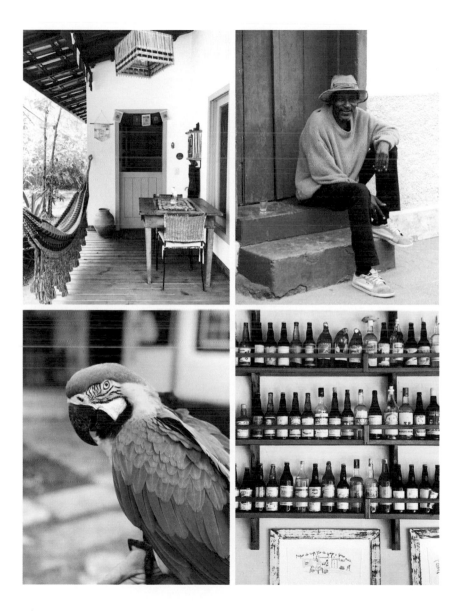

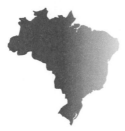

I HAD ALWAYS THOUGHT of myself as a person who prioritized family time more than most, but then my cousin Alicia moved to Brazil and . . . I changed my mind. As part of her PhD in political science, Alicia spent five years doing fieldwork in Ceará, in the northeast part of the country, and I began to feel vicarious exhaustion just *listening* to her talk about the spirited scene down there. "We think *our* family is close," she'd say, "but you should see these Brazilian families, man. They're basically always together. No alone time. And they love to celebrate."

I have a large extended family myself, with about thirty aunts and uncles and twenty first cousins, and I genuinely enjoy hanging out with all of them—so my "no thank you" reaction to constant togetherness surprised me. But understand: While Alicia was doing a large chunk of her fieldwork, I was living by myself in a small studio apartment on the Upper West Side in Manhattan. I was all about "working on myself" during those years. The scene in Brazil sounded a bit overwhelming in comparison—suffocating, even. When did Brazilians do their random wandering? When did they self-reflect? Every morning,

I woke up at 7:30 a.m. to go running in Central Park, and I tried to write in my journal at night with a glass of red wine as often as I could. My editors knew that I loved all things self-actualization, so they gave me lots of magazine assignments in that realm of thinking, too, from finding happiness within, to the power of setting boundaries. I *loved* my me-time at home, my time when I didn't have to answer to anyone, my time when I could just shuffle around the apartment doing weird solo things, like standing in front of the fridge in my sports bra eating a can of refried beans with a spoon.

But then the *New York Times* published an op-ed called "Happiness Is Other People" that prompted me to reassess my thinking and look at Alicia's descriptions of Brazil in a new light. In it, the author, Ruth Whippman—a Brit who moved to America and then wrote *America the Anxious*—argued that the biggest problem with happiness in America is that it's considered a largely solitary pursuit. She highlighted the absolute irony of the fact that we Americans have created an entire industry around the idea that happiness comes from within, but the truth is that an overwhelming amount of research continues to prove that happiness usually comes from the outside, in the form of in-person social connections.

That's exactly why I decided to include Brazil in this book. Whippman ultimately helped me realize that we may have it all backwards, that *I'd* maybe had it all backwards. "Self-reflection, introspection, and some degree of solitude are important parts of a psychologically healthy life," she wrote in her op-ed. "But somewhere along the line we seem to have gotten the balance wrong." Could getting a feel for Brazil's celebratory, close-knit

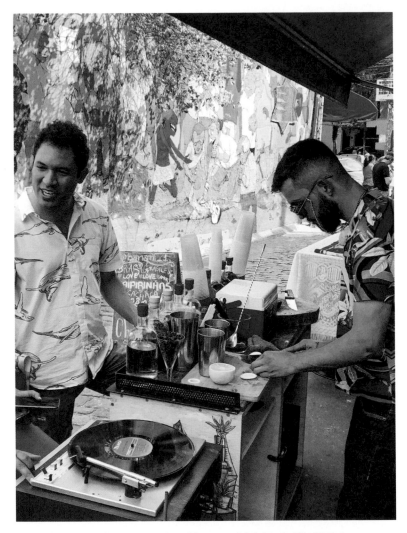

São Paulo: A street vendor whips up caipirinhas in Vila Madalena,
a lively neighborhood known for its street art.

culture help inspire me, and us, to shift the balance back to the other side?

As a travel journalist, I knew that Brazil isn't a super popular destination with American tourists. Even though many Americans love and dream about Carnaval and are quite obsessed with Brazilian soccer, the truth is that the majority of travelers still tend to head elsewhere when they fly south: to Peru for the Andes, perhaps; to Argentina for the Malbec; to Chile for the Patagonia adventures. Brazil is home to 206 million people, yet only 6.6 million travelers visit each year. Part of that low number is Brazil's reputation; many Americans think the favelas (low-income and marginalized neighborhoods in the big cities), for example, are simply too dangerous to take the risk. But some of it is also the tourism infrastructure itself. Up until June 2018, Americans had to apply for a visa to enter the country, which influenced many travelers to go someplace easier.

No matter the exact reason, I thought it was even more important to include Brazil in this book precisely *because* it isn't as well traveled. It's not exactly known as a typical "wellness" destination, either, at least not like a Tulum or a Bali. I knew there were pockets of traditionally "healthy" vibes, particularly in Rio, where locals play volleyball on the beach or exercise in one of the city's popular outdoor gyms, and then replenish themselves with a fresh coconut or an açai bowl for good measure. But in many other parts of the country, it's a lot of fried food and heavy meat, especially in the southern regions of the country (the north is more seafood heavy).

From what I'd heard, though, well-being in Brazil isn't really about the food, at least not from a cultural standpoint. It's generally about the people. To investigate this idea even further, my plan was to fly into São Paulo and then make my way to the southeastern state of Minas Gerais first, followed by Bahia—another one of Brazil's twenty-six states—on the northeastern coast. I first learned about Minas Gerais at a media event after I'd started telling some members of one of Brazil's tourism associations about my book idea. I told them that I was inspired by Whippman's op-ed and thought that I could expand on that idea in my own research. One woman, Nadja Hofmann—a German living in Brazil—told me I *had* to visit her in the state of Minas Gerais. She said visiting her there would be perfect for my book: We would attend a big community party at a 12,000-acre farm commune, and then we would hang out with her adopted Brazilian family (more on that later). Then, for the second leg of my trip, Alicia had told me that there's a large "hammock culture" in the northeast part of the country, in which communities spend a significant portion of their day hanging out in hammocks on their front porches or at the beach—and I thought that was as good a place as any to learn even more about Brazil's cultural connectedness.

When most people think of Brazil, they tend to think of Carnaval, coconuts, colors, and caipirinhas, the country's national cocktail made with cachaça (a local Brazilian liquor that, similar to rum, is made from fermented sugarcane juice) and sugar and lime. I quickly learned that my first stop,

Minas Gerais——just Minas for short——is not really any of those things.

As a landlocked interior state known for its sweeping rolling hills, its lush farms, its abundance of cheese, and its coffee production (it's the leading coffee state in Brazil), Minas remains largely off the tourist map, beloved by Brazilians, yet mostly unknown to foreigners. When the late Anthony Bourdain traveled there for his globe-trotting show *Parts Unknown*, he confirmed my in-the-dark experience: "Chances are, you've never been here. In fact, it's likely that you've never even heard of this place. But if you travel through Brazil and you talk about food, which I have and I do, you hear about this place. You hear about it seemingly a lot."

I reached the entrance to the farm commune, called the Comuna do Ibitipoca, around 10 p.m. on a Thursday night in

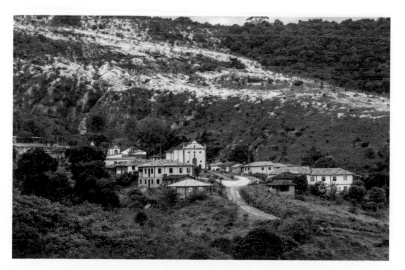

Minas Gerais: La Comuna, where the party took place, was straight out of a storybook!

December. Sitting in the back seat, I heard the gravel crunching slowly underneath the car wheels as we made our way up the long driveway, and I was riddled with anticipation. Is there any better feeling in the world than arriving in a new destination and wondering? You have no idea what the air will smell like, or who you will meet at a cute corner bar, or if you will have a life-changing revelation. Soon you'll develop a favorite drink order, and you'll taste that one street food that you won't be able to stop dreaming about for years, and you'll meet that person who you now know was *meant* to enter into your life at that exact time on that exact trip. But in that moment, it's just you and your unknowns, you and your curiosity for what will be. I *live* for that excitement.

When the car finally stopped, a young Brazilian man in khakis was waiting for me by the door with a bright blue and yellow toucan perched on his shoulder. "Come in, come in," he called as I got out of the car. The stars were shining brightly overhead, tons of them, and I could hear the crickets chirping. This was the kind of place that helps you put your worries in perspective. "I'm Rodrigo, the manager here, and this is Antônio. Don't worry, he's super friendly," he assured me as he stroked Antônio's feathers and led me inside.

The whole place smelled like a bonfire. There were two wood-burning stoves, cozy sheepskin rugs in the hallways, and gorgeous artworks featuring natural settings on the walls. Made entirely from reclaimed wood, the pousada—the Portuguese word for a boutique inn—had eight suites, a dining area, a small outdoor bar with twinkly lights hanging from the wooden beams, and a yoga hut a couple feet away. "This doesn't exactly seem like the place for a raging party," I laughed to Rodrigo before heading into my room for the night.

"Oh, don't worry," he replied with a knowing grin. "This is only the beginning. The party is going to be epic. You just wait."

In the morning, I met the owner of the commune, Renato Machado, for breakfast. He had a kind, dad-like demeanor and salt-and-pepper hair that reminded me of a Brazilian George Clooney. Over coffee and pão de queijo—traditional Brazilian cheese bread made from cassava flour and local cheese—I learned that the near-sixty-year-old bought the 12,000 acres of deforested rolling hills back in the 1980s, and has taken it upon himself to bring the land back to life. Today, nearly 90 percent of the trees on his land have grown back thanks to his reforestation efforts, and travelers now stay in wooden guest cabins scattered around all of this property, in addition to the main pousada. But he was quick to tell me that he didn't reforest the land alone. He built an entire community in and around his property, one focused entirely on sustainability—and that was going to be the community gathering for the party.

For the record, I was slightly nervous about attending this celebration, as I would hardly know anyone and I didn't speak the language minus the few Portuguese phrases I'd learned in prep for my trip. ("Eu não falo português"—"I don't speak Portuguese"—was particularly helpful.) But once I met Renato and some other members of the community on my first morning, I felt so welcome, and I knew I'd be okay for the big bash the next day.

TURNS OUT, BRAZILIAN PARTIES LIVE UP TO THE HYPE. The festivities kicked off around 9:30 a.m. with coffee and pão de queijo for breakfast again. (Though pão de queijo is found all over Brazil, it originated in Minas, so some people there claim it's the best in the country.) The highlight after that was watching a group of incredibly fit Brazilians perform capoeira, an Afro-Brazilian martial art that began as a resistance movement and combines dancing, music, and acrobatics. Once that performance was over, one of Renato's friends, Paulo, a real estate consultant in his mid-fifties who'd traveled to Minas from Rio for the party, saw me standing by myself for a moment and brought me into a dance group that had just formed. "It's time to learn how to dance samba," he told me.

As a well-documented jam band fan, my preferred method of dancing is the kind you see at Phish shows, where you sort of just nod your head to the beat, swing your hips every so often, and occasionally stare at the sky. It's a very low-maintenance, unstructured kind of movement, and does not require any advance planning or knowledge of any variety. Samba, on the other hand, has actual formal steps, and I wanted to do my best to learn them since the dance is such an important part of Brazilian culture. Its roots trace all the way back to the enslaved West African people in Bahia who were brought to the country by Portuguese traders. Like many groups of enslaved people around the world, they turned to music and dance as a way to express their feelings, whether those feelings were painful or hopeful or spiritual or all of the above. Samba today has come to define the spirit of Carnaval, representing a unified racial and social spirit in a land once divided by slavery, and it's also been exported around the world. And yet! Despite wanting to honor this cultural history so very badly, I was so very bad at actually mastering the moves.

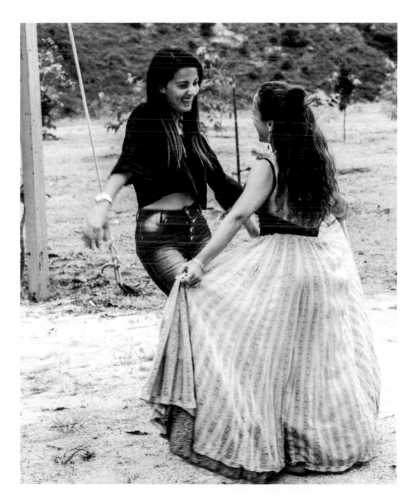

Minas Gerais: These women were samba goals.

The History of Celebration in Brazil

As Paulo said, Brazilians certainly know how to party. But not everything is cheer and cachaça. Like many countries with a devastating history, Brazil's spirit of celebration is deeply rooted in colonization and slavery. It's important to keep this past in mind to understand the full context of its present. Here's a brief timeline:

1500: The Portuguese arrived in Brazil.

1530: The Portuguese began to import enslaved African people to Brazil, having founded the Atlantic slave trade in the 1450s. In part because Brazil was closer to Africa than the Caribbean and North America, slavery in Brazil became entrenched incredibly quickly.

1822: Brazil declared independence from Portugal, but maintained slavery. This is in large part because it was Portugal's crown prince who declared Brazil's independence from Portugal—and then crowned himself Emperor because he didn't want to return to Portugal to rule. So even though Brazil was no longer a colony, it was still ruled by the same Portuguese elite. Slavery continued to be so ingrained in the culture that it was hardly even challenged until 1873, when writer and advocate Joaquim Nabuco formed the Anti-Slavery Society in the hopes of ending slavery in Brazil.

1888: Brazil finally abolished slavery, officially becoming the last nation in the Western hemisphere to do so. At that point, an estimated 4.5 million enslaved people had been transported from Africa—roughly a third of the total number taken to the Americas. Enslaved people had become the largest population in Brazil.

1888-PRESENT DAY: More than three hundred years of slavery left Brazil racially and socially divided, with an incredibly long history of social, economic, and political inequality that the country still struggles with to this day. Nearly 25 percent of Brazil's population lives below the poverty line, and the majority of these residents are descendants of former enslaved people. Celebrations have come to represent a release from the ongoing ramifications of this divided past. During Carnaval, Brazilians wear masks and, if only for a little while, cultural barriers cease to exist and the country is unified. That spirit seeps into Brazilian life throughout the rest of the year, too, in which moments of celebration are often the only respite from a hard life.

"Do you dance all that often in New York?" Paulo laughed as I fumbled my way around. (I had a flashback to my hiking guide in Norway asking me if I had ever hiked before, and began to pick up on an embarrassing running theme.)

"Yeah, I do . . . but not really in such a structured way, I guess," I laughed, thinking of my classic flowy Phish sway.

Paulo was nice enough to continue as my partner for a couple more songs, bless his heart, and then he brought me over to his friends, who welcomed me into the group with open arms. We spent the rest of the afternoon into the night snacking on pastéis (crispy, deep-fried dough filled with meat, cheese, or hearts of palm) and coxinha (shredded chicken and mashed potatoes smothered in bread crumbs and deep-fried), and drinking Brahma (a local Brazilian beer) and cachaça straight with no chaser. Most of the group didn't speak English, so we had all sorts of fun conversations through Google Translate:

Me: I'm sorry I'm bad at Portuguese!

Him/her: I'm sorry I'm bad at English!

Me: It's okay, let's drink more cachaça!

Everyone, laughing: Yes! Saúde! (Cheers!)

And so it went.

"We give a lot of value for leisure here in Brazil," Paulo told me at one point, gesturing around. "We think that if you're really well but you work a lot, what's the point? Even the poor, they work and they have fun. We run on this sense that we all have good things and bad things in our lives, but we celebrate together no matter what," he continued. "Fun is very important here—it's a big part of being well. Just look at this party! It's a huge part of our culture."

After the party, it was time to meet up with Nadja and her adopted family. "It's not really adopted in the way that you may think of adoption as an American," she'd clarified back in New York. "But that's what they call it in Brazil." She'd met a woman named Célia at a bar in the local town near the commune, and Célia invited her to come over for dinner with her family. "Then she asked me to come again the next day, and soon enough, she was asking me to spend the night, too," Nadja continued. As more and more time went by, Nadja found herself at Célia's house nearly every day before and after her volunteer work, which soon turned into salaried work, and she was learning Portuguese and feeling happier than she ever had. Pretty soon she moved in, and now she's a member of the family. Just like that. "It's a very Brazilian thing to do, to take care of someone like that as if they were your own," she told me.

She wasn't kidding. After my trip, I called Cláudio Torres, PhD, a professor at the Institute of Psychology at the University of Brasília who studies the nuances of Brazilian culture, to go over some of the lessons I learned in Brazil while I was there. And he confirmed that, in Brazil, your family is not just your parents and your siblings—and it's not even just your blood relatives. Your family includes everyone from your aunts and your uncles to your cousins and even your friends. Your family includes that neighbor who has lived next door to you your whole life, or your mom or your dad's work partner that's always at your house. "All of those people, no matter how close they are to you by blood, can voice their opinions in pretty much the same way your parents can." Brazilians can even be members of multiple different families at the same time, because other families, as a general rule, can take you in as their own. "You just need one person in the family to introduce you," Cláudio told me. "And then, if they deem you trustworthy and think you are a good person and you share the same values as they do, you're part of the family forever—provided you continue to follow the family rules."

Nadja's adopted Brazilian family lives in São José dos Lopes, a tiny village in the municipality of Lima Duarte with only three main streets and about a hundred houses total. It's a twenty-minute drive from the Comuna's main pousada, where I stayed when I was there. There's one bar, which Nadja's Brazilian dad, Domingus, owns and operates every night (he works in the fields during the day), plus a hospital, a school, and a community center that Renato built for the locals. And that's it. Back in New York, Nadja had told me that São José dos Lopes is the kind of place that sucks you in and steals your heart and makes you never want to leave, and on the day I went to meet her family, I could feel what she meant right away. The town felt welcoming in the way that only small villages can, like you're stepping into the equivalent of that bar where everyone knows your name.

Nadja and Célia were waiting outside their house to greet me and her brother Junior, who had driven me over from the Comuna, where he works (remember, many people in the villages surrounding Renato's land are affiliated with the Comuna in some way). Célia gave me a giant welcome hug and two kisses on each cheek—the customary greeting in Brazil, known as *beijinhos* (little kisses)—and motioned for me to head inside.

"She's so excited to meet you but nervous that you won't like the food," Nadja whispered in my ear as we walked, although she didn't *really* need to whisper because her mom doesn't speak English. "She keeps saying it's just 'simple food' and is afraid that you won't like it because it isn't fancy." I'm definitely not the fancy type, but I was coming from New York City, and to her, that may have meant luxury. I told Nadja to tell her that I love home-cooked food, and that I'm so grateful to her for making it for me. Célia smiled and immediately relaxed once she received this translation, and we were on our way.

The lunch was delicious, of course, perhaps my favorite meal that I ate my entire time in Brazil. Célia had prepared rice and beans, which most Brazilians eat every day, plus pulled pork, zucchini, farofa (toasted cassava flour), and corn bread, all to be washed down with a huge glass of ice-cold Coke. But of course it wasn't about the lunch. When is the lunch ever really about the lunch? It was about the laughter and the warmth that took place around the table. Domingus had even come home from the fields, where he keeps thirty-six cows, to eat together and to meet me. While we were all sitting there chowing down, two neighbors popped into the kitchen, as is often the case in their small village, and the whole table started cracking up after the second one, Marquinho, apparently said that I was pretty and could he buy me a watch.

"That's so typical of him!" they all laughed.

"What a flirt!"

"Welcome to life in São José dos Lopes!"

And the laughter didn't stop throughout the lunch. Somehow, even though I don't speak Portuguese and Nadja

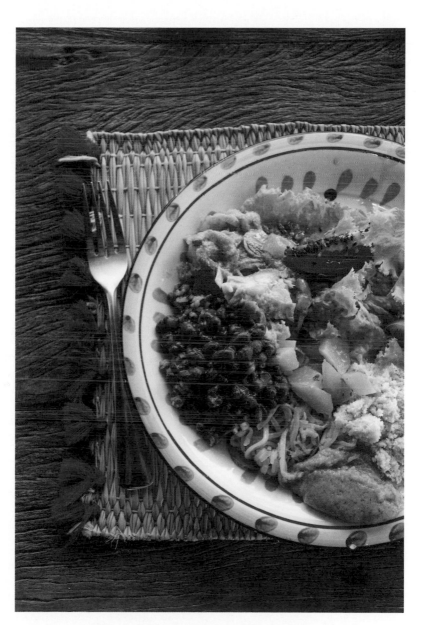

Bahia: In Brazil, sharing your meals with others is
often just as important as the food itself.

was translating everything, we all had a blast, just sitting and enjoying each other's company, cracking up at the hilarity of the watch situation and at how I ate so much more than Nadja did. (It was seriously flavorful, especially the juicy pulled pork. And I also knew from having an Indian mother-in-law that eating a mother's home-cooked food is a great way to show your thanks, especially when you can't communicate all that well otherwise.)

It didn't take long for Célia to tell me that she wanted me to stay for more time.

"Told you," Nadja smiled knowingly.

I shook my head and said that I'd love to stay but I had to get home to my life in New York soon, at which point Célia got very serious. The reason she took Nadja in, she explained, is that her son, Junior, left to study in Oakland, California, for three months in 2014—and those three months were the longest months of her entire life. She missed him so much and so deeply, a longing Brazilians refer to as *saudade*. "I told myself that I would always take care of anyone who came my way, because I spent so much time wishing someone was taking care of him while he was away," she told me. Couldn't she take care of me? Célia's sentiment was so sweet, I wanted to cry. And for many Brazilians, that's the whole point of saudade—they just want to feel. They *love* feeling. Feeling brings them joy.

———

After lunch, Nadja took me for a stroll around the village, just the two of us, and told me that that constant hangout time with her Brazilian family has meant more to her than most people know.

Embrace Your Emotions with Saudade

Saudade is one of those words that Brazilians say can't be directly translated into English, but the gist is that it's the emotional pain that comes from missing someone or something you love. Here's a brief breakdown:

THE ROOT MEANING: *Saudade* comes from the Spanish word *solidad*, which translates to "solitude" in English—meaning it used to be about being alone after someone or everyone has left you.

ITS EVERYDAY USE: "Nowadays, Brazilians use *saudade* for everything, not just people," Cláudio told me after my trip. One of his coworkers who studied in the US said he even feels saudade for Starbucks!

Yet although saudade is about a sad feeling, it also brings Brazilians lots of happiness at the same time. "It has a good part, too, because it means that you love someone, and it's always good to love someone in the end, even if they're gone," Cláudio continued. "It's a strange train of thoughts, but it's very important to us. Most Brazilians are proud to say that the word *saudade* only exists in Portuguese."

THE BIGGER PICTURE: Saudade speaks to the utter importance Brazilians place on community. Their emphasis on connection is so strong that they have an entire *word* for missing someone so much it hurts.

And while people often mistake the concept of saudade for Brazil's answer to nostalgia, it's not that, not really at all. Nostalgia is when you feel sad for something that will never be back again, whereas you can feel saudade for someone or something that will be back again at a future point. There's even an added layer in which people get anxious about wanting to "kill their saudade" and just hang out already.

"The need to kill our saudade makes us hang out together even more because we really look forward to matando saudade ('killing saudade')," Cláudio explained. How cool is it that the Brazilian emphasis on hanging out is so strong that a general anxiety tends to develop when you are *not* able to hang out?

In fact, it has helped her heal. Back in Germany, she struggled with depression all throughout college, at times not leaving her bed for days. All she wanted to do was crawl into a hole and be alone. But when she started living in São José dos Lopes, there was no such possibility. Her family was always around, because, in her experience, "You can never be alone when you're part of a Brazilian family—someone always wants to be in your presence." And you know what happened? Her depression lifted a little bit. "What happens here is that everyone just pulls you in so you can't escape. And at some point, I can't pinpoint exactly when, I realized that I actually didn't *want* to escape—I felt better when I was surrounded by people who loved me," she continued. "My tendency is to want alone time, but I realized that, for the first time in my life, I didn't want to be alone. Being around a community of people helped me feel so much better."

Of course, this is just one person's story. And not all Brazilian families are like a warm hug.

But still, at the same time, most Brazilians have a strong network of people they know they can rely on, whether that's friends or family. A 2019 study about Brazilian culture found that Brazilians' entire identity is "derived mainly from the immediate and extended family, where individuals have strong social ties with their social groups, especially family, and prefer to make group decisions in general." Another Brazilian I spoke with before my trip, Alicia's friend José, told me that he's in a WhatsApp group with sixty of his family members—yes, sixty!—and they make the time to say good morning to each other every single day when they wake up. All sixty of them. The group also shares links to funny videos and articles throughout the day, and José says that if you don't respond to everything, you're in for it, man: "If you don't say 'good morning' each day, or you stop reacting to the links, someone will inevitably call you out and say, 'Hey! You're not reacting! Is everything okay?' It's nuts."

Can you even imagine? Saying good morning to sixty of your nearest and dearest, every morning? I have a hard time keeping up with my family group texts that have *eight* people in them, let alone adding some serious double digits. But ultimately, José's love for his family overrides his frustrations. "Brazilians love to connect and we love to share, which is why we love WhatsApp so much," he told me with a laugh. (It's true: While WhatsApp is popular in many countries around the world, Brazil uses the platform the most, with India coming in at number two.)

ACCORDING TO CLÁUDIO, FAMILY STRUCTURE IN BRAZIL PLAYS THE BIGGEST ROLE IN OVERALL WELL-BEING.

"Brazilian families are literally the center of Brazilian society," he said. To illustrate this point, he told me a story. A couple years after his parents moved from Rio to Brasília when he was young, his mother got sick with cancer. Rather than go to the hospital in Brasília, it was decided by the whole family that she needed to go back to Rio to get her care there. "She needed to be in the center of our family, because she couldn't get well without being around everyone—that's how strong our ties are," he explained.

In the end, Cláudio told me, that's the crucial difference between wellness in the States and wellness in Brazil: It's more of a group effort in the latter. "From my experience as a Brazilian

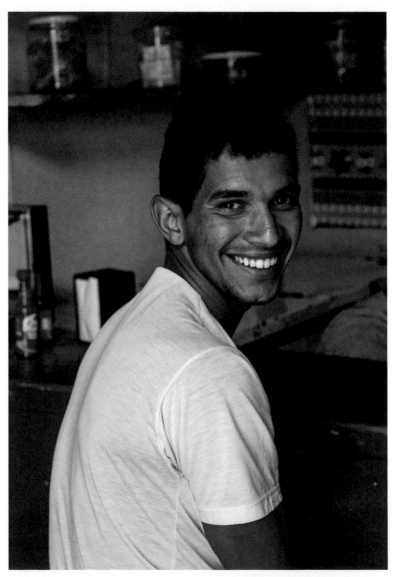
Minas Gerais: Many Brazilians like Junior understand that their own well-being is directly tied to their family's well-being.

who lived in the United States for five years, I found that wellness in America is about yourself: If you're healthy physically and psychologically, if you're financially well, if you're in a good relationship, and if you eat well, you're considered healthy in the public eye. But while Brazilians of course care about those things, too, the biggest factor of all is your family—you cannot be well if your family is not well. Well-being is a group thing, not an individual thing. Just being around everyone is the best way to feel well."

There are lots of families in the United States that join together when things get rough, too. But while there isn't concrete data to support this feeling, many say anecdotally that that philosophy simply isn't as entrenched in the States. One woman I got introduced to through the Brazilian grapevine, an American teacher who lives in Boston but spends her summers living in northeast Brazil, told me that "there's a general loyalty that exists within Brazil that I don't tend to see on the same level in the US. We have pockets of close family and friend groups, of course, but not as consistently. It's just so tight-knit in Brazil all the time—families mean the world to each other."

And in the end, isn't that the whole thing? Many Brazilians intuitively understand the value of hanging out as a wellness practice. A 2015 study published in the *American Journal of Lifestyle Medicine* even gave this idea a name: the *connection prescription*. Its authors write that social connection is a pillar of lifestyle medicine: "Humans are wired to connect," they write in the study, "and this connection affects our health. From psychological theories to recent research, there is significant evidence that social support and feeling connected can help people maintain a healthy body-mass index, control blood sugars, improve cancer survival, decrease cardiovascular mortality, decrease depressive symptoms, mitigate post-traumatic stress disorder symptoms, and improve overall mental health."

This communal support is a basic truth to many Brazilians. They know what it's like to lean on each other in times of need. Alicia's friend Blaise, a social- and environmental-policy consultant who lives in Rio, put it best: "Lives here are more unstable than in other parts of the world, jobs are lost, people don't have insurance or savings, and people are basically poorer in general. Everyone is aware of that reality, and that's what brings people together, too, this idea that you need to help each other through tough times, because everyone will go through it at some point or another."

"DO YOU SIT IN A HAMMOCK EVERY DAY?" I ASKED MY NEW BRAZILIAN FRIEND JOAQUIM AS I WAS LOOKING UP AT THE MOON.

It was my second night on the Maraú Peninsula in southern Bahia, one of the nine states in northeast Brazil and my final stop. I was staying at a family-run bohemian guest lodge right on the beach, where Joaquim and his mom and stepdad run the show. While I had spent some time exploring the town and wandering the beach that day, I'd spent *most* of my time hammock hopping in the name of research—and I wanted to get Joaquim's take on the northeastern hammock culture I'd heard so much about.

"Of course I sit in the hammock every day," he replied with a laugh. *How is that even a question?* his eyes seemed to ask. If you lived in a tropical hideaway by the beach, wouldn't you?

"The hammock is one of the greatest inventions of all time," he continued. "Every day after work I just chill, lie in the hammock, and do some swinging. It's the best way to relax, just sitting in there. It's hard to get out, you know? Don't disturb me please, I'm in the hammock. I'm gone."

Two years ago, Joaquim left his friends and the rest of his family in Rio, where he grew up, to come north to Bahia to live

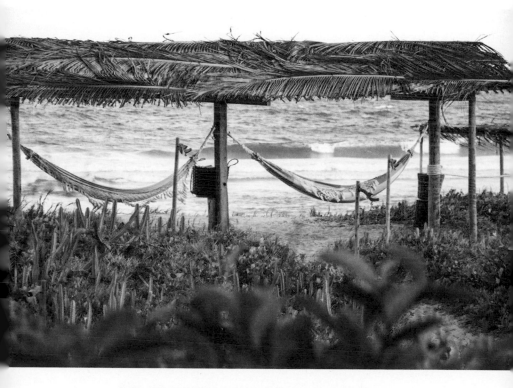

Bahia: Who wouldn't want to hang in that hammock?

with and work for his mom and stepdad, who'd opened the lodge in 2013. Throughout my trip, I'd learned that in Brazil, living with and working for your parents is perfectly normal. In fact, unlike in the US, where living with your parents is sometimes— though not always—painted as some sort of career or maturity failure, Brazilian parents are all too pleased when their kids boomerang back to them. They *want* their kids back. Most never wanted them to leave in the first place. One of my taxi drivers in São Paulo told me that he thinks of his family as one big "safety net," always there to ease the pain of daily life. His kids are eighteen, twenty-two, and twenty-six, and they all still live with him. "I'm just happier when we're all in the same room— it's as simple as that," he said.

But still, I wondered if Joaquim felt a sense of saudade for his friends and the rest of his family back in Rio. When I was twenty-five, I was working as an associate editor at a women's magazine, going to media events or out with friends nearly every night. I was all city, all friends, all the time—did he miss that?

"Oh, every day," he answered within seconds of my asking. "I talk to my friends and family every day on WhatsApp, but then I see them making plans in all of my WhatsApp groups, and I miss them so much. I feel such a sense of saudade that I'm not there to go out to that bar that they're all going to, or to congratulate my friend for being with the girl he likes."

Like most humans who reflect on their big life choices, Joaquim then told me he's in a constant state of indecision, weighing the pros and cons of his life choice to chill in Bahia. On the one hand, his physical body is quite pleased with his laid-back beachfront day-to-day. He's getting more sleep, and he's eating a lot better, too, a result of not succumbing to the conveniences of urban living (aka takeout and the restaurant scene). But on the other hand, he sees other families chilling at home in their hammocks, and it makes him miss his nearest and dearest even more.

"My body is technically 'healthy' here," he said, placing air quotes around the word. "But I don't know if I'm healthy overall. We Brazilians are so emotional, and I think that we feel our feelings more deeply than other people do—so I get very sad about missing my friends and the rest of my family in Rio and not having a girlfriend," he continued. "That sadness also helps me appreciate them more, and I remind myself that this is a choice that I made to live out here, too, but still . . . we'll see."

And that, in a (Brazil) nutshell, is what I love the most about Brazilians, or at least the ones I met: They understand the importance of community. The fact that Joaquim was so quick to include his community in his evaluation of his overall well-being was not lost on me. It tracked with everything I'd learned from all of the other Brazilians and adopted Brazilians I'd met along the way, from Alicia to José to Nadja to Paulo and more. They all focused on the big thing first: the people. It's always the people in the end. It's the people who make your world. And sitting there in that hammock, listening to Joaquim prioritize his friends and family first, I took a deep breath of ocean air and smiled—because I was finally going back home to my own.

Hang Out Like a Brazilian...

WHEREVER YOU ARE

Honor your social commitments.

We often think of wellness as a solitary pursuit, like taking a bubble bath. But really, human connection comes above all else, and we should all be treating our relationships in a way that reflects that. Next time you feel like bailing on a happy hour or that birthday party, whether it's virtual or in person, try reframing it as a dedication to your overall health instead.

Lean into the group text.

I probably won't start texting my entire extended family good morning when I wake up. But it couldn't hurt to put in a bit more effort. Dip your toe in: If you're on WhatsApp, start a few new groups devoted to particular subjects, and see what happens.

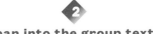

Leisure time is sacred. Treat it accordingly.

I see you, person who is "watching Netflix" while texting and replying to emails, and cooking dinner in between. Multitasking can be okay at work, but it defeats the purpose of relaxing! Practice the art of lying on your bed and staring at the ceiling, doing absolutely nothing at all.

Feel deeply.

Many Brazilians see missing someone as a natural part of life, one that reminds them of the deep love they feel for someone who's absent in their current day-to-day. To feel this distinctly Brazilian and Portuguese emotion yourself, scroll through your social media posts or page through old albums for photographs of someone you love. Instead of feeling sad about the people you miss, try to reframe the narrative and remind yourself that you're happy you have such strong, loving feelings for your people in the first place.

Get a hammock.

Stress reducing and super comfortable, they may actually be one of the greatest inventions of all time. If you live in an urban area and don't have room in your house, a portable outdoor hammock is a good compromise.

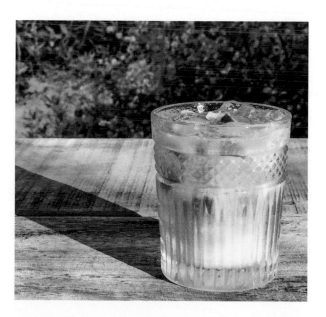

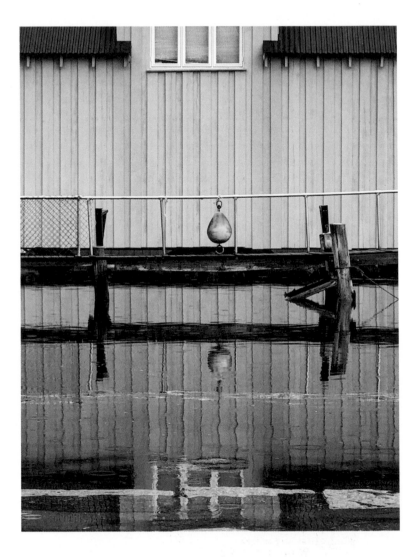

Grounded

WRAPPED UP MY final trip for this book in December 2019 and handed in the first draft of this manuscript about a month later, just weeks before COVID-19 grounded the globe—which means I can't stop thinking about the cosmic timing of this book. What if I'd started it just a little bit later? What if I'd planned to do all of my research at the beginning of 2020? What if I'd gotten sick on the road? This book would not exist. So now, I am all the more grateful that it does.

I'm currently writing to you from my brother's friend's house in Charlottesville, Virginia, where Rahul and I came to ride out the pandemic away from its epicenter in New York. We are so fortunate to have had the option to leave Brooklyn, and in many ways, the wisdom I gathered while reporting this book has been the key to helping us feel okay during this surreal time.

Like many people around the world, Rahul and I have taken to cooking up a storm, leaning on fresh dishes I learned about on my travels, like Ital stew and Kerala-inspired coconut curry, to keep us feeling healthy and balanced. Inspired by Norwegian friluftsliv, we've gone on a nature walk most nights after work, strolling next to the nearby river and taking the time to smell the sweet lilac blossoms blooming on its bank. In an effort to incorporate more of Ayurveda's grounding dinacharya rituals into our daily routines, we've tried to go to bed and wake up just a little bit earlier, and have successfully started each day with a glass of warm water before diving into the coffee pot. Faced with so much uncertainty in the future, both our own and the world's, we've taken comfort in the Hawaiian philosophy that we don't have to have it all planned out, that our life roadmap will reveal itself to us in due time. We've leaned into the stillness, too, into the quiet that surprised me with its sweetness in the Japanese countryside, occasionally even choosing to wake up to the peaceful sound of the birds rather than my standard "morning tunes" playlists.

And man, have we connected. For a while there, it was Zoom or bust. In true Brazilian style, we've both spent more time talking on the phone with our people than we have in years. My WhatsApp has been blowing up, too, filled with just-checking-in messages from those I've met on my travels. If there's one silver lining to all of this, one bright light hidden in the darkness, it's that our world has gotten both smaller and bigger at the same time. While our day-to-day excursions have been reduced to walking by the river behind our house and going grocery shopping, our focus and our outlook has expanded, widened, and grown more global than ever.

AT FIRST, I THOUGHT IT MIGHT BE STRANGE TO REVISE AND EDIT THIS BOOK DURING THIS PANDEMIC. It felt jarring to go from a life of constant motion to a life of constant stillness, and I wasn't sure how that sharp lurch would impact my mental state as I spent time reflecting on my initial words. Would the editing process rub salt into the wound? Would I find myself longing for the road and for the freedom I found there, longing for the times that were? Fortunately, I realized pretty quickly into the work that my answers were no, no, and no. If anything, taking the advice I gathered during this time has proven that it's advice worth taking.

I know that feeling good during a pandemic is rooted in privilege. Low-income Americans and people of color are dying at a disproportionate rate, with many unable to say goodbye to their loved ones. The economy has plummeted, and it will be incredibly difficult to recover from its devastating economic impact for decades to come. Jobs, relationships, and other timely life events have been put on hold indefinitely. Even the Hawaiians on Maunakea had to take down their base camp, leaving the outcome of their peaceful demonstrations uncertain. Ultimately, having the time to even *think* about well-being during this time is a luxury, one I don't take for granted. That's why I feel incredibly grateful to be among those who have been able to take this time to reevaluate our lives. After all, as the air has become cleaner and the normally murky Venice canals have cleared up and mountain goats have even been spotted wandering the streets of a town in North Wales, people have started to notice how badly Mother Nature needed this reset. As life has come to an abrupt standstill, people have begun to see what beauty there can be in slowing down.

I love travel so much. It's part of who I am. I love how it gives people the opportunity to connect and to inspire and to learn and to grow. But reflecting on the lessons I learned through a pandemic lens confirmed that we don't even need to travel to put them to use in our daily lives. At the time the manuscript for this book went to print, the world was still mostly on lockdown, and the future of travel remained uncertain. I'm hopeful that it will resume at some point, and that it will come back even better than it was before: more sustainable, more inclusive, and more kind. I'm also hopeful that the communities around the world who rely on tourism to survive will recover from this massive blow. But in the meantime, I'm happy to discover that all of the advice I gathered on the road truly applies *wherever you are*. At least I certainly think it does. And I also take comfort in the fact that these lessons got me through some of the darkest times I've ever experienced—so I can only imagine they'll still hold true when the world brightens up once again.

Acknowledgments

TO MY AMAZING EDITOR, Cara Bedick: Thank you for getting my vision for this book right away, and for your wisdom and patience as we moved it through all of its various stages. I knew I was in good, smart hands the whole time, and your confidence in me also made me more confident in myself.

Thank you to my wonderful agent, Sarah Smith, for believing in me and this book from Day One. Remember when *Destination Wellness* was just an email and a life dream? We did it. I'm so happy and grateful that you were on this mission with me.

To the talented team at Chronicle Prism, especially Mark Tauber, Jenn Jensen, and Pamela Geismar: You went above and beyond! Thank you for showering *Destination Wellness* with all of your TLC. You only publish your first book once, and I'm honored that I got to publish mine with you.

Thank you to my hosts in each destination: to Chris and Lisa Binns, Mark and Alecia Swainbank, Empress Thandi, and Michael Gordon for sharing your Rastafari knowledge; to the Visitors Bureau and the Four Seasons in Hawai'i, especially Crissa Hiranaga, Yvonne Hunter, Lori Holland, Alli Adams, Anna Piergallini, Shere'e Quitevis, and Pua Sterling, for showering me with aloha; to Exodus Travel, especially Britney Hope, for sending me on a dream trip to Japan and taking care of me when I almost got trapped by the typhoon; to Tom Lund and crew, for welcoming me into your chosen family in Sogndal; to Ragnhild, for taking me in as your own; to Innovation Norway, for your help and support; to the staff at Nattika in Kerala, for sharing your wisdom so generously; to the Brazilian Luxury Tourism Association, for taking me under your wing.

Thank you to both of my parents for your unconditional love and for teaching me early on that words matter. To my mom: You will always be Editor Mom. Thank you for reading a million drafts and for helping me give them their shape. I know that both they and I "sparkle plenty" because of you. To my dad: Your constant "My daughter is writing a book! How did I get so lucky?" texts got me through this process. Thank you for always reminding me to zoom out, but also for making time to zoom in on all of the little details with me—your edits and our heady chats made this book infinitely better.

Tom and Meg, you are the coolest and most supportive siblings around. TAM forever. And to our newest addition, Jessica Manly: We're so happy to have you in the family. Thanks to my stepdad Steve, for your upbeat nature and constant encouragement. And to my stepmom Anne, for your everlasting warmth and cheer.

Big O and Joann, I hope I'm still traveling well into my nineties like you are! Your dedication to adventure and to family inspires me to no end. Neelam, Rajesh, and Priya—where to begin? I feel so lucky to call you my family. Thank you for teaching me that your home in New Delhi is my home now, too.

Big hugs to Lindsay Maitland Hunt, for your unwavering belief that this is a book that needs to be out there in the world. *Destination Wellness* would not exist without you.

Huge thanks to Jo Piazza, for telling me in your oh-so-Jo way: "You should be a travel writer." Here I am, and I will remain forever grateful to you for your guidance and encouragement.

To Shannon Rosenberg, Amanda Schupak, John Dioso, Jahlani Niaah, Jake Homiak, Scott Saft, Claudio Torres, Shigenori Nagamoto, and Vishwanath Guddadar: Thank you for your sharp eyes and edits, and for caring about me and my book so very much.

Thank you to my wonderful community for showing up for me throughout this book process. As usual, Dylan says it best: "I'd be lost if not for you." To my never-peaking Dickinson women (Miri Goodman, Zoë Stopak-Behr, Julie Hunter, Kate McMullen), and my huge family on all sides (Dalys, Healys, and Khoslas), and Jack Coulton, Cecilia Estreich, Sarah Vaynerman, Bonnie Glass, Carrie Greig, Courtney Lynn, Jason-Louise Graham, Amy Gordon, Katie Distelrath, Laura Biffar, Vicki Fulop, Jess Simmons, Sara Olchowski, Abbe Wright, Lauren Oster, Kafi Drexel, Janet Siroto, Marnie Schwartz, Sam Cassetty, Leah Ginsberg, Alex Diaz, Stacey Lindsay, Jess Dailey, Sophie Friedman, Devin Tomb, Malia Griggs, Paul Jebara, David Jefferys, Monica Mendal, and Christine Byrne: Your support means the world.

And finally, to Rahul. Thank you for inspiring me to take a chance on myself. Your entrepreneurial confidence has definitely rubbed off on me. I could not have written this book without your endless support, your relentless positivity, and your ability to set aside your FOMO to encourage me to travel the world solo. I love you so much, and I can't wait to travel together once again.

REFERENCES

Before Takeoff

Global Wellness Institute. *Global Wellness Economy Monitor*, 2018. https://globalwellnessinstitute.org/industry-research/2018-global -wellness-economy-monitor/

Happiness Research Institute. *Wellbeing Adjusted Life Years: A Universal Metric to Quantify the Happiness Return on Investment*, April 2020. https://6e3636b7-ad2f-4292-b910-faa23b9c20aa.filesusr .com/ugd/928487_1595c32a127341f7a2769c624898dc6c.pdf

Larocca, Amy. "In a Pandemic, Is 'Wellness' Just Being Well-off?" The Cut. April 2020. https://www.thecut.com/2020/04/wellness -during-coronavirus.html

United Nations. *World Happiness Report*, 2019. https://world happiness.report/ed/2019/

JAMAICA: Ital Is Vital

Afari, Yasus. *Overstanding Rastafari: Jamaica's Gift to the World.* Senya-Cum, 2007.

Dickerson, Mandy Garner. "I-tal Foodways: Nourishing Rastafarian bodies." Louisiana State University & Agricultural and Mechanical College. LSU Master's Thesis, 2004.

Gonsalves, Mama T. *Ital Is Vital, 365 Days a Year.* Amazon.com Services LLC: Kindle Edition, January 30, 2018.

Jaffe, Rivke. "Ital Chic: Rastafari, Resistance, and the Politics of Consumption in Jamaica." *Small Axe: A Caribbean Journal of Criticism*, March 1, 2010.

Tantamango-Bartley, Yessenia. "Vegetarian Diets and the Incidence of Cancer in a Low-Risk Population." *Cancer Epidemiology, Biomarkers & Prevention,* February 2013. https://www.ncbi.nlm.nih.gov/pmc/articles /PMC3565018/

West, Brett J. "The Potential Health Benefits of Noni Juice: A Review of Human Intervention Studies." *Foods*, April 11, 2018. https://www.ncbi.nlm.nih.gov/pmc/articles/PMC5920423/

Yuajah, Empress. *Rasta Way of Life: Rastafari Livity Book*. Self-published, 2014.

NORWAY: Get Outside

Associated Press. "Brazilian surfer rides 80-foot wave off Portugal, new world record." May 2018. https://globalnews.ca/news/4178438 /brazilian-surfer-80-foot-wave-world-record/

Gordon, Amie M. "6 Ways to Find Awe in Your Everyday Life." *Psychology Today*. September 30, 2015. https://www.psychology today.com/us/blog/between-you-and-me/201509/6-ways-find-awe -in-your-everyday-life

Greater Good Science Center at UC Berkeley. "The Science of Awe." September 2018. https://ggsc.berkeley.edu/images/uploads /GGSC-JTF_White_Paper-Awe_FINAL.pdf

Hartig, Terri, PhD. Professor of Environmental Psychology in Sweden. Phone interview, April 30, 2020.

Hofmann, Annette R., Carsten Gade Rolland, Kolbjørn Rafoss, and Herbert Zoglowek. *Norwegian Friluftsliv: A Way of Living and Learning in Nature*. Münster: Waxmann, 2019.

United States Environmental Protection Agency. *Report on the Environment: Indoor Air Quality*, July 16, 2018. https://www.epa.gov /report-environment/indoor-air-quality

Williams, Kathryn, PhD. Professor of Environmental Psychology in Australia. Email interview, April 30, 2020.

HAWAIʻI: Nānā I Ke Kumu (Look to the Source)

Aha Punana Leo. "A Timeline of Revitalization." https://www .ahapunanaleo.org/new-page-2

Goo, Sara Kehaulani. "The Hawaiian Language Nearly Died. A Radio Show Sparked Its Revival." *Code Switch*. NPR, June 22, 2019. https://www.npr.org/sections/codeswitch/2019/06/22/452551172 /the-hawaiian-language-nearly-died-a-radio-show-sparked-its-revival

McCann, Adam. "Happiest States in America." WalletHub, September 9, 2019. https://wallethub.com/edu/happiest-states /6959/

Pukui, Mary Kawena, E. W. Haertig MD, and Catherine A.Lee. *Nānā I Ke Kumu (Look to the Source).* Vol. I. Honolulu: Hui Hānai, 1972.

JAPAN: Be Present

García, Héctor, and Francesc Miralles. *The Book of Ichigo Ichie: The Art of Making the Most of Every Moment, the Japanese Way.* New York: Penguin Books, 2019.

Jordan, Alec. "Christel Takigawa: Looking into Tokyo's Olympic Future." *Tokyo Weekender,* November 17, 2013. https://www.tokyo weekender.com/2013/11/christel-takigawa-looking-into-tokyos -olympic-future/

Kumai, Candace. *Kintsugi Wellness: The Japanese Art of Nourishing Mind, Body, and Spirit.* New York: HarperCollins Publishers, 2018.

Longhurst, Erin Niimi. *A Little Book of Japanese Contentments: Ikigai, Forest Bathing, Wabi-sabi, and More.* San Francisco: Chronicle Books, 2018.

Otake, Tomoko. "1 in 4 Firms in Japan Say Workers Log over 80 Overtime Hours a Month." *The Japan Times,* October 7, 2016. https://www.japantimes.co.jp/news/2016/10/07/national/social -issues/1-in-4-firms-say-some-workers-log-80-hours-overtime-a -month-white-paper-on-karoshi/#.XwyrBpNKjfY

INDIA: Make It Personal with Ayurveda

Ajmera, Ananta Ripa. *The Ayurveda Way: 108 Practices from the World's Oldest Healing System for Better Sleep, Less Stress, Optimal Digestion, and More.* North Adams, MA: Storey Publishing, 2017.

Bhattacharya, Dr. Bhaswati. *Everyday Ayurveda: Daily Habits That Can Change Your Life.* Gurgaon: Penguin Random House India, 2015.

Casperson, Erin. Dean of the Kripalu School of Ayurveda. Zoom interview, April 15, 2020.

ET Bureau. "77 Percent Indian Households Use Ayurvedic Products: PwC report." *The Economic Times (India Times),* November 23, 2018. https://economictimes.indiatimes.com/industry/healthcare /biotech/healthcare/77-percent-indian-households-use-ayurvedic -products-pwc-report/articleshow/66773295.cms?from=mdr

Lad, Vasant, BAMS, MASc. *Ayurveda: The Science of Self-Healing. A Practical Guide.* Twin Lakes: Lotus Press, 1985.

Lad, Vasant, BAMS, MASc. *The Complete Book of Ayurvedic Home Remedies: Based on the Timeless Wisdom of India's 5,000-Year-Old Medical System.* New York: Harmony, 1999.

National Family Health Survey, India, 2016. http://rchiips.org/nfhs /NFHS-4Report.shtml

Pushpanath, Salim, Jacob Philip, and Dr. Vijayachandradas. *Essential Ayurveda.* Kerala: Dee Bee Info Publications, 2005.

BRAZIL: Embrace Your Community

Dessen, M. A., and C. V. Torres. "Family and Socialization Factors in Brazil: An Overview." *Online Readings in Psychology and Culture,* 2019. https://doi.org/10.9707/2307-0919.1060

Martino, Jessica, Jennifer Pegg, Elizabeth Pegg Frates, MD. "The Connection Prescription: Using the Power of Social Interactions and the Deep Desire for Connectedness to Empower Health and Wellness." *The American Journal of Lifestyle Medicine,* October 7, 2015. https://www.ncbi.nlm.nih.gov/pmc/articles/PMC6125010/

Rodgers, Carly. "The Paradox of Carnaval." Think Brazil, February 27, 2018. https://www.wilsoncenter.org/blog post/the-paradox -carnaval-afro-brazilian-contributions-to-national-celebration

Torres, Cláudio V. "A Meta-Analysis of Basic Human Values in Brazil: Observed Differences within the Country." Brazilian Association of Organizational and Work Psychology. 2015. http://pepsic.bvsalud. org/scielo.php?script=sci_arttext&pid=S1984-66572015000100009

Whippman, Ruth. "Happiness Is Other People." *New York Times,* October 27, 2017. https://www.nytimes.com/2017/10/27/opinion /sunday/happiness-is-other-people.html

ABOUT THE AUTHOR

ANNIE DALY is a fourth-generation freelance journalist. A former editor at *Self, Yahoo! Travel, BuzzFeed Travel, Cosmopolitan*, and *Good Housekeeping,* she has written for *Afar, Condé Nast Traveler*, and more. She lives in New York City with her husband.